Alzheimer's Diet Cookbook and Guide

for the Newly Diagnosed

Simple, Healthy Recipes, Key Insights, and a 28-Day Meal Plan for Early Alzheimer's Management

Judy Kelly

Copyright © Judy Kelly, 2024.

All rights reserved. No part of this publication may be reproduced, distributed, or transmitted in any form or by any means, including photocopying, recording, or other electronic or mechanical methods, without the prior written permission of the publisher, except in the case of brief quotations embodied in critical reviews and certain other noncommercial uses permitted by copyright law.

Table of Contents

1. **Introduction**   3
   - Understanding Alzheimer's Disease Understanding Alzheimer's Disease   5
   - Importance of Diet in Alzheimer's Management   8
   - How to Use This Cookbook   11
2. **Getting Started**   14
   - Stocking Your Pantry: Essential Ingredients   14
   - Kitchen Tools and Equipment   16
   - Tips for Meal Planning and Preparation   18
3. **Brain-Boosting Nutrients**   20
   - Key Nutrients for Cognitive Health   20
   - Foods to Include and Avoid for Cognitive Health   22
4. **Breakfast Recipes**   25
5. **Lunch Recipes**   36
6. **Dinner Recipes**   50
7. **Snacks and Appetizers**   68
8. **Desserts**   78
9. **28-Day Meal Plan**   91
10. **Lifestyle Tips**   107
    Hydration and Brain Health   107
    Physical Activity and Cognitive Function   108
    Stress Management and Sleep   109
11. **Conclusion**   111

1. Introduction

Welcome to the "Alzheimer's Diet Cookbook and Guide for the Newly Diagnosed." If you or a loved one has recently received an Alzheimer's diagnosis, you may be experiencing a whirlwind of emotions—fear, confusion, and uncertainty about the future. It's natural to feel overwhelmed, but remember, you are not alone. This book is here to support you on this journey.

Alzheimer's disease affects millions of people worldwide, and while there is no cure, there are ways to manage symptoms and improve quality of life. One of the most powerful tools at your disposal is nutrition. A well-balanced diet can play a crucial role in supporting brain health, enhancing cognitive function, and promoting overall well-being.

This cookbook and guide have been carefully crafted with you in mind. We've included simple, healthy recipes that are not only delicious but also packed with nutrients known to benefit the brain. You'll find a variety of meals that cater to different tastes and dietary needs, ensuring you can enjoy a diverse and satisfying diet.

Beyond the recipes, this book provides key insights into the role of nutrition in managing Alzheimer's. You'll learn about essential nutrients, foods to include and avoid, and practical tips for meal planning and preparation. We've also included a 28-day meal plan to help you get started, complete with weekly shopping lists and easy-to-follow recipes.

We understand that living with Alzheimer's can be challenging, and caring for someone with the disease can be equally demanding. That's why we've included lifestyle tips to help you manage stress, stay hydrated, and incorporate physical activity into your routine. Our goal is to empower you with the knowledge and tools you need to take control of your health and make informed choices.

As you embark on this journey, remember that small, consistent changes can make a big difference. Take things one step at a time, and don't hesitate to seek support from friends, family, and healthcare professionals. This book is just one resource among many, and together, we can navigate this path with hope and resilience.

Thank you for choosing this guide. We hope it brings you comfort, encouragement, and practical advice as you take steps towards a healthier, more fulfilling life. Remember, you are not alone in this journey—we are here with you every step of the way.

With warmth and empathy,
Judy Kelly

- Understanding Alzheimer's Disease Understanding Alzheimer's Disease

Alzheimer's disease is a complex and challenging condition that affects millions of people around the world. It's the most common form of dementia, a general term for memory loss and other cognitive impairments that interfere with daily life. Understanding the basics of Alzheimer's can help you navigate the journey ahead with greater confidence and clarity.

What is Alzheimer's Disease?

Alzheimer's disease is a progressive neurological disorder that leads to the degeneration and death of brain cells. It affects memory, thinking, behavior, and the ability to perform everyday tasks. The disease typically progresses slowly, beginning with mild memory loss and eventually leading to severe cognitive decline and the inability to communicate or respond to the environment.

Symptoms of Alzheimer's Disease

The symptoms of Alzheimer's can vary from person to person, but they generally follow a similar pattern as the disease progresses:

1. Early-Stage (Mild) Alzheimer's:
    - Memory loss, especially of recent events or information
    - Difficulty with problem-solving or planning
    - Challenges with completing familiar tasks
    - Confusion about time or place
    - Trouble finding the right words or understanding visual images

2. Middle-Stage (Moderate) Alzheimer's:
    - Increased memory loss and confusion
    - Difficulty recognizing family and friends
    - Repetitive statements or questions
    - Wandering or getting lost
    - Personality and behavior changes, such as increased irritability or aggression

3. Late-Stage (Severe) Alzheimer's:
   - Severe memory loss and cognitive decline
   - Inability to communicate coherently
   - Need for full-time assistance with daily activities
   - Physical decline, including difficulty swallowing and mobility issues

Causes and Risk Factors

The exact cause of Alzheimer's disease is not fully understood, but it is believed to result from a combination of genetic, environmental, and lifestyle factors. Some key factors that may increase the risk of developing Alzheimer's include:

- Age: The risk increases significantly after age 65.
- Family History: Having a parent or sibling with Alzheimer's increases your risk.
- Genetics: Certain genes are associated with an increased risk.
- Head Injuries: A history of severe head trauma may be linked to Alzheimer's.
- Heart Health: Conditions that damage the heart or blood vessels, such as high blood pressure, diabetes, and high cholesterol, may increase the risk.

Importance of Early Diagnosis

Early diagnosis of Alzheimer's disease is crucial for several reasons:

- Planning and Preparation: It allows individuals and their families to plan for the future, make important decisions, and arrange for necessary care.
- Management of Symptoms: Early intervention can help manage symptoms and improve quality of life through medications, lifestyle changes, and supportive therapies.
- Access to Resources: An early diagnosis provides access to resources, support groups, and clinical trials that may offer additional support and treatment options.

The Role of Diet and Lifestyle

While there is no cure for Alzheimer's, research suggests that diet and lifestyle can play a significant role in managing the disease and potentially slowing its progression. A diet rich in brain-boosting nutrients, regular physical activity, mental stimulation, and social engagement are all important factors in maintaining cognitive health.

In this book, we will explore how a balanced, nutritious diet can support brain health and provide practical recipes and tips to help you or your loved one live a healthier, more fulfilling life despite the challenges of Alzheimer's disease.

Remember, understanding Alzheimer's is the first step in taking control of your health and well-being. As you continue reading, you'll find valuable information and resources to guide you on this journey.

- Importance of Diet in Alzheimer's Management

The relationship between diet and cognitive health has been the subject of extensive research, revealing that what we eat can significantly influence brain function and overall well-being. For those diagnosed with Alzheimer's disease, adopting a nutritious diet can be a powerful tool in managing symptoms and potentially slowing the progression of the disease.

Brain-Boosting Nutrients

Certain nutrients are particularly beneficial for brain health. Including these in your diet can help support cognitive function and reduce inflammation, which is linked to Alzheimer's. Key brain-boosting nutrients include:

- Omega-3 Fatty Acids: Found in fatty fish (like salmon, mackerel, and sardines), flaxseeds, chia seeds, and walnuts, omega-3s are essential for brain health and can help reduce inflammation.
- Antioxidants: Foods rich in antioxidants, such as berries, dark chocolate, nuts, and colorful vegetables, help combat oxidative stress and protect brain cells.
- B Vitamins: Vitamins B6, B12, and folate play crucial roles in brain function and can be found in leafy greens, whole grains, legumes, and fortified cereals.
- Vitamin E: Nuts, seeds, spinach, and broccoli are excellent sources of vitamin E, an antioxidant that may help protect brain cells from damage.
- Polyphenols: These compounds, found in tea, coffee, red wine (in moderation), and various fruits and vegetables, have been shown to support brain health.

Benefits of a Healthy Diet for Alzheimer's Patients

1. Enhanced Cognitive Function: A diet rich in brain-boosting nutrients can help improve memory, focus, and overall cognitive performance.
2. Reduced Inflammation: Chronic inflammation is linked to many neurodegenerative diseases, including Alzheimer's. Anti-inflammatory foods, such as fruits, vegetables, and fatty fish, can help reduce inflammation in the brain.

3. Better Heart Health: A healthy diet supports cardiovascular health, which is closely linked to brain health. Improved blood flow and reduced risk of heart disease can positively impact cognitive function.

4. Weight Management: Maintaining a healthy weight is important for overall well-being and can help prevent other health issues that may exacerbate Alzheimer's symptoms.

5. Improved Mood and Energy Levels: Nutrient-dense foods provide the energy and nutrients needed to maintain a positive mood and high energy levels, which can be particularly beneficial for those managing Alzheimer's.

Dietary Patterns for Alzheimer's Management

Several dietary patterns have been studied for their potential benefits in managing Alzheimer's disease. Incorporating elements from these diets can be a practical approach:

- Mediterranean Diet: Emphasizes fruits, vegetables, whole grains, legumes, nuts, seeds, fish, and olive oil, with moderate consumption of dairy and limited red meat.
- DASH Diet: Designed to lower blood pressure, the DASH diet focuses on fruits, vegetables, whole grains, lean proteins, and low-fat dairy, while limiting salt, sugar, and red meat.
- MIND Diet: A hybrid of the Mediterranean and DASH diets, the MIND diet specifically targets brain health, encouraging the consumption of green leafy vegetables, berries, nuts, whole grains, fish, poultry, beans, and olive oil, while limiting red meat, butter, cheese, pastries, and fried foods.

Practical Tips for Incorporating a Healthy Diet

1. Plan Your Meals: Take the time to plan balanced meals that include a variety of brain-boosting foods. This can help ensure you're getting the necessary nutrients.
2. Stay Hydrated: Proper hydration is essential for cognitive function. Aim to drink plenty of water throughout the day.
3. Limit Processed Foods: Reduce your intake of processed foods, which are often high in unhealthy fats, sugars, and salt, and can negatively impact brain health.

4. Focus on Fresh Ingredients: Choose fresh, whole foods whenever possible to maximize nutrient intake and minimize exposure to additives and preservatives.
5. Moderation is Key: While it's important to focus on healthy eating, it's also crucial to enjoy your food and allow for occasional treats in moderation.

Incorporating these dietary strategies can help you take an active role in managing Alzheimer's disease. While diet alone cannot cure or completely prevent Alzheimer's, it is a valuable component of a comprehensive approach to treatment and care. By making informed choices about what you eat, you can support your brain health and improve your quality of life.

- How to Use This Cookbook

Welcome to the "Alzheimer's Diet Cookbook and Guide for the Newly Diagnosed." This book is designed to be a practical and supportive resource as you navigate life with Alzheimer's disease. Whether you are newly diagnosed, caring for someone with the disease, or simply looking to support brain health through nutrition, this cookbook will provide you with valuable information, delicious recipes, and practical tips. Here's how to get the most out of this book:

Navigating the Sections

1. Introduction and Understanding Alzheimer's Disease
   - Begin with these sections to gain a fundamental understanding of Alzheimer's disease, its symptoms, and its progression. This knowledge will help you appreciate the importance of diet in managing the disease.

2. Getting Started
   - This section provides essential information on setting up your kitchen for success. Learn about the key ingredients and tools you'll need to prepare the recipes in this book, along with tips for meal planning and preparation.

3. Brain-Boosting Nutrients
   - Familiarize yourself with the nutrients that support cognitive health. This section explains the role of various nutrients and guides you on incorporating them into your daily diet.

4. Recipes
   - The heart of the book, this section is divided into breakfast, lunch, dinner, snacks, appetizers, and desserts. Each recipe is designed to be simple, healthy, and beneficial for brain health. Follow the clear instructions and use the provided tips to make cooking enjoyable and stress-free.

5. 28-Day Meal Plan
   - The 28-day meal plan is a structured guide to help you get started on your journey to better nutrition. Each week includes a shopping list and a selection of

recipes from the book. Use this plan to simplify meal planning and ensure a balanced, nutrient-rich diet.

6. Lifestyle Tips
   - Beyond diet, this section offers practical advice on hydration, physical activity, stress management, and sleep. These tips will help you create a holistic approach to managing Alzheimer's.

Making the Most of the Recipes

- Follow the Instructions: Each recipe is designed to be easy to follow. Read through the instructions before you start cooking to ensure you understand each step.
- Adapt to Your Needs: Feel free to adapt recipes to suit your tastes and dietary needs. If you have any specific dietary restrictions, consult with a healthcare professional to make appropriate substitutions.
- Use Fresh Ingredients: Whenever possible, use fresh, high-quality ingredients to maximize the nutritional value and flavor of your meals.
- Meal Prep and Batch Cooking: Consider preparing larger batches of meals and storing leftovers for later use. This can save time and ensure you always have healthy options available.

Engaging with the Meal Plan

- Weekly Shopping Lists: Use the provided shopping lists to simplify your grocery trips. Having all the necessary ingredients on hand will make cooking more convenient and enjoyable.
- Stay Flexible: The meal plan is a guide, not a strict regimen. Feel free to swap recipes or adjust portions to fit your preferences and lifestyle.
- Monitor Progress: Keep track of how different foods and meals make you feel. Note any changes in energy levels, mood, or cognitive function, and adjust your diet accordingly.

Incorporating Lifestyle Tips

- Hydrate Regularly: Aim to drink plenty of water throughout the day. Proper hydration is essential for overall health and cognitive function.
- Stay Active: Incorporate physical activity into your daily routine. Even gentle exercises like walking or stretching can have significant benefits.
- Manage Stress: Practice stress-reducing techniques such as meditation, deep breathing, or spending time in nature.
- Prioritize Sleep: Aim for consistent, quality sleep each night. Establish a bedtime routine and create a restful sleep environment.

Seeking Support

- Engage with Communities: Join support groups or online communities for individuals and caregivers affected by Alzheimer's. Sharing experiences and tips can provide emotional support and practical advice.
- Consult Professionals: Regularly consult with healthcare professionals, including doctors, nutritionists, and therapists, to ensure you are following the best possible care plan.

We hope this cookbook becomes a trusted companion on your journey to better health and well-being. Remember, every small step you take towards a healthier lifestyle can make a meaningful difference. Thank you for choosing this guide, and we wish you the best on your path to managing Alzheimer's with compassion and resilience.

2. Getting Started

- Stocking Your Pantry: Essential Ingredients

Setting up your pantry with essential ingredients is the first step towards creating nutritious and delicious meals that support brain health. Here's a guide to stocking your pantry with key items for the recipes in this cookbook:

1. Grains and Legumes
- Whole grains such as brown rice, quinoa, oats, and whole wheat pasta
- Legumes like lentils, chickpeas, black beans, and kidney beans

2. Fruits and Vegetables
- Fresh fruits such as berries, apples, oranges, and bananas
- Leafy greens like spinach, kale, and arugula
- Cruciferous vegetables including broccoli, cauliflower, and Brussels sprouts

3. Lean Proteins
- Lean cuts of poultry such as chicken breast and turkey
- Fatty fish rich in omega-3s like salmon, mackerel, and trout
- Plant-based proteins such as tofu, tempeh, and edamame

4. Healthy Fats
- Extra virgin olive oil for cooking and salad dressings
- Avocados for adding creamy texture and healthy fats
- Nuts and seeds such as almonds, walnuts, chia seeds, and flaxseeds

5. Dairy and Alternatives
- Low-fat dairy products like yogurt and milk (if tolerated)
- Non-dairy alternatives such as almond milk or soy yogurt

6. Herbs, Spices, and Flavor Enhancers
- Fresh herbs like parsley, cilantro, basil, and mint
- Spices such as turmeric, cinnamon, ginger, and garlic powder
- Low-sodium vegetable or chicken broth for adding flavor to soups and stews

7. Sweeteners and Condiments
- Natural sweeteners like honey or maple syrup (use sparingly)
- Low-sodium soy sauce or tamari for seasoning
- Mustard, vinegar, and lemon juice for marinades and dressings

8. Whole Food Snacks
- Whole grain crackers or rice cakes for quick snacks
- Popcorn kernels for a healthy, homemade snack
- Dried fruits like apricots, raisins, or cranberries for a sweet treat

Tips for Organizing Your Pantry
- Label and Date: Keep items organized and labeled, and rotate them to use older items first.
- Keep It Visible: Store healthier options at eye level for easy access and visibility.
- Minimize Processed Foods: Limit the presence of processed and sugary snacks to encourage healthier choices.

By stocking your pantry with these essential ingredients, you'll have everything you need to prepare nourishing meals that support brain health and overall well-being. These ingredients form the foundation of the recipes in this cookbook, ensuring you can create delicious dishes with ease. Adjust your pantry to accommodate any dietary preferences or restrictions, and enjoy exploring the variety of flavors and nutrients that support a healthier lifestyle.

- Kitchen Tools and Equipment

Equipping your kitchen with the right tools and equipment can make meal preparation easier and more enjoyable. Here's a guide to essential kitchen tools you'll need for cooking the recipes in this cookbook:

1. Cookware
- Non-Stick Skillet: Ideal for cooking eggs, pancakes, and sautéing vegetables with minimal oil.
- Saucepan: Used for boiling grains, making sauces, and heating soups.
- Stockpot: Essential for cooking large batches of soups, stews, and pasta dishes.
- Baking Sheet: Used for roasting vegetables or baking dishes like casseroles.

2. Knives and Cutting Tools
- Chef's Knife: A versatile knife for chopping, slicing, and mincing vegetables, fruits, and meats.
- Paring Knife: Useful for detailed tasks like peeling fruits or trimming vegetables.
- Cutting Board: Provides a stable surface for chopping ingredients without damaging your countertops.

3. Food Prep Essentials
- Mixing Bowls: Various sizes for mixing ingredients, marinating, and storing leftovers.
- Measuring Cups and Spoons: Accurately measure liquids, dry ingredients, and spices for precise cooking.
- Colander or Strainer: Used for draining pasta, rinsing vegetables, or washing fruits.

4. Small Appliances
- Blender or Food Processor: Essential for making smoothies, sauces, and pureeing ingredients.
- Toaster or Toaster Oven: For toasting bread, reheating leftovers, or baking small dishes.
- Slow Cooker or Instant Pot: Convenient for preparing soups, stews, and one-pot meals with minimal effort.

5. Utensils
- Wooden Spoon and Spatula: Gentle on cookware and ideal for stirring sauces and sautéing.
- Tongs: Useful for flipping foods on the grill or in the oven, and serving salads.
- Whisk: Essential for blending ingredients smoothly and incorporating air into batters.

6. Baking and Cooking Accessories
- Oven Mitts or Pot Holders: Protect hands from heat when handling hot cookware or baking dishes.
- Silicone Baking Mats or Parchment Paper: Prevents sticking when baking cookies or roasting vegetables.
- Kitchen Timer: Helps you keep track of cooking times for multiple dishes.

7. Storage and Organization
- Food Storage Containers: Store leftovers or prepared ingredients for future meals.
- Reusable Bags or Wraps: Reduce waste by storing food items like sandwiches or snacks.

Tips for Organizing Your Kitchen
- Declutter Regularly: Keep countertops clear and organize cabinets to easily access frequently used items.
- Clean as You Cook: Maintain a clean workspace by washing dishes, wiping counters, and putting away ingredients as you cook.
- Invest in Quality: Choose durable and versatile tools that will last and enhance your cooking experience.

By equipping your kitchen with these essential tools and equipment, you'll be well-prepared to tackle the recipes in this cookbook with confidence and efficiency. Enjoy the process of cooking nutritious meals that support brain health and overall well-being!

- Tips for Meal Planning and Preparation

Meal planning and preparation are essential for maintaining a healthy diet, especially when managing Alzheimer's disease. Here are practical tips to help you streamline your meal planning process and make cooking more efficient:

1. Set Aside Dedicated Time
- Designate a specific day each week for meal planning and grocery shopping. This routine helps you stay organized and ensures you have everything you need for the week ahead.

2. Create a Weekly Menu
- Plan your meals for the week, including breakfasts, lunches, dinners, and snacks. Refer to the recipes in this cookbook for inspiration and variety.
- Consider dietary preferences, nutritional needs, and portion sizes when selecting recipes.

3. Make a Shopping List
- Based on your menu, create a detailed shopping list of ingredients you'll need for each meal. Organize your list by categories (e.g., produce, dairy, pantry items) to streamline your shopping trip.

4. Stock Up on Staples
- Keep essential pantry items and ingredients stocked, such as grains, legumes, spices, and cooking oils. This ensures you can quickly whip up meals without needing to make frequent grocery runs.

5. Prep Ingredients in Advance
- Wash, chop, and portion out ingredients ahead of time, such as vegetables, fruits, and proteins. Store them in air-tight containers or zip-top bags for easy access during meal preparation.

6. Utilize Batch Cooking- Cook larger quantities of meals and portion them into individual servings. This method saves time and ensures you have ready-to-eat meals available throughout the week.

7. Consider Freezing Meals
- Some recipes can be prepared in advance and frozen for later use. Label and date containers or bags to easily identify meals and ensure freshness.

8. Use Time-Saving Cooking Methods
- Opt for quick and efficient cooking methods like stir-frying, sheet pan roasting, or using a slow cooker or Instant Pot. These methods require minimal hands-on time while delivering delicious results.

9. Stay Flexible
- Be adaptable with your meal plan and recipes. Adjust based on ingredients you have on hand or changes in your schedule.

10. Involve Others
- Cooking can be a social activity. Invite family members or caregivers to join you in meal preparation, making it a bonding experience.

11. Monitor and Adjust
- Pay attention to how meals impact energy levels, mood, and cognitive function. Adjust your meal plan and recipes as needed to support overall well-being.

12. Enjoy the Process
- Embrace the opportunity to nourish yourself or your loved one with nutritious and flavorful meals. Cooking can be therapeutic and enjoyable, enhancing both physical and mental health.

By incorporating these meal planning and preparation tips into your routine, you can simplify the process of cooking healthy meals while managing Alzheimer's disease. With careful planning and organization, you'll be able to maintain a balanced diet that supports brain health and overall well-being.

3. Brain-Boosting Nutrients

- Key Nutrients for Cognitive Health

Maintaining cognitive health is crucial, especially for individuals managing Alzheimer's disease. Incorporating the following key nutrients into your diet can support brain function and overall well-being:

1. Omega-3 Fatty Acids
- Sources: Fatty fish (such as salmon, mackerel, and sardines), flaxseeds, chia seeds, walnuts.
- Benefits: Omega-3s are essential for brain health, supporting cognitive function and potentially reducing inflammation in the brain.

2. Antioxidants
- Sources: Berries (like blueberries, strawberries, and raspberries), dark chocolate (in moderation), nuts (such as almonds and walnuts), colorful vegetables (like spinach, kale, and beets).
- Benefits: Antioxidants help protect brain cells from oxidative stress and may improve cognitive performance.

3. B Vitamins
- Sources: Leafy greens (such as spinach and kale), whole grains (like brown rice and oats), legumes (including lentils and chickpeas), fortified cereals.
- Benefits: B vitamins (particularly B6, B12, and folate) play a role in cognitive function, supporting memory and mood regulation.

4. Vitamin E
- Sources: Nuts and seeds (such as almonds and sunflower seeds), spinach, broccoli, avocado.
- Benefits: Vitamin E is an antioxidant that may help protect nerve cells and support overall brain health.

5. Polyphenols
- Sources: Tea (green and black), red wine (in moderation), dark chocolate, fruits (like berries and apples), vegetables (such as spinach and broccoli).
- Benefits: Polyphenols have anti-inflammatory properties and may help improve cognitive function and protect against neurodegenerative diseases.

6. Vitamin D
- Sources: Fatty fish (like salmon and tuna), fortified dairy products (milk and yogurt), egg yolks, sunlight exposure.
- Benefits: Vitamin D plays a role in brain health and may reduce the risk of cognitive decline.

7. Magnesium
- Sources: Leafy greens (such as spinach and Swiss chard), nuts and seeds (like almonds and pumpkin seeds), whole grains (including quinoa and brown rice).
- Benefits: Magnesium supports cognitive function and helps regulate neurotransmitter pathways in the brain.

8. Zinc
- Sources: Shellfish (such as oysters and shrimp), lean meats (like beef and chicken), nuts (including cashews and almonds), legumes (such as lentils and chickpeas).
- Benefits: Zinc is involved in neurotransmission and may support memory and learning processes.

9. Water
- Sources: Watermelon, cucumber, spinach, green beans, coffee, herbal tea, tofu

- Foods to Include and Avoid for Cognitive Health

Maintaining a diet that supports cognitive health is crucial, especially for individuals managing Alzheimer's disease. Here are guidelines on foods to include and avoid:

Foods to Include:

1. Fatty Fish: Salmon, mackerel, trout, and sardines are rich in omega-3 fatty acids, which are essential for brain health.

2. Berries: Blueberries, strawberries, and raspberries are packed with antioxidants that help protect brain cells from damage.

3. Leafy Greens: Spinach, kale, and collard greens are high in vitamins, minerals, and antioxidants that support cognitive function.

4. Nuts and Seeds: Walnuts, almonds, flaxseeds, and chia seeds provide omega-3s, antioxidants, and vitamin E, beneficial for brain health.

5. Whole Grains: Brown rice, oats, quinoa, and whole wheat are rich in fiber and B vitamins, supporting brain function.

6. Lean Proteins: Chicken, turkey, tofu, and beans provide essential amino acids for neurotransmitter function and overall brain health.

7. Colorful Vegetables: Bell peppers, tomatoes, and carrots contain antioxidants and nutrients that support cognitive function.

8. Legumes: Lentils, chickpeas, and black beans are rich in protein, fiber, and folate, beneficial for brain health.

9. Healthy Fats: Olive oil, avocado, and nuts provide monounsaturated fats and vitamin E, supporting brain function.

10. Herbs and Spices: Turmeric, cinnamon, and ginger have anti-inflammatory properties that may benefit brain health.

Foods to Avoid or Limit:

1. Processed Foods: Reduce consumption of processed snacks, fast food, and sugary treats, which offer little nutritional benefit and may contribute to inflammation.

2. Saturated and Trans Fats: Limit intake of red meat, butter, and full-fat dairy, as well as foods containing trans fats (partially hydrogenated oils), which can negatively impact heart and brain health.

3. Added Sugars: Minimize consumption of sugary beverages, candies, and desserts, as high sugar intake may impair cognitive function and increase inflammation.

4. Highly Salted Foods: Excess sodium can contribute to high blood pressure, which may negatively affect brain health over time.

5. Alcohol: Limit alcohol consumption, as excessive intake can impair cognitive function and overall brain health.

6. Artificial Sweeteners: Some research suggests that artificial sweeteners may impact gut health, which can influence cognitive function indirectly.

7. Highly Processed Meats: Reduce consumption of processed meats such as bacon, sausage, and deli meats, which may contain additives and preservatives linked to inflammation.

General Tips:

- Stay Hydrated: Drink plenty of water throughout the day to support overall health, including brain function.

- Balance Meals: Aim for balanced meals that include a variety of nutrients from different food groups.
- Moderation: Enjoy treats and less healthy foods in moderation while focusing on a diet rich in whole, nutrient-dense foods.

By incorporating these guidelines into your diet, you can support cognitive health and overall well-being while managing Alzheimer's disease. Consult with a healthcare professional or registered dietitian for personalized advice and guidance based on individual health needs and preferences.

4. Breakfast Recipes

1. Blueberry Almond Overnight Oats

Ingredients:
- 1/2 cup rolled oats
- 1/2 cup almond milk
- 1/4 cup Greek yogurt
- 1/4 cup fresh blueberries
- 1 tablespoon almond butter
- 1 tablespoon chia seeds
- Optional: honey or maple syrup for sweetness

Instructions:
1. In a jar or bowl, combine rolled oats, almond milk, Greek yogurt, almond butter, and chia seeds.
2. Stir well to mix all ingredients evenly.
3. Gently fold in fresh blueberries.
4. Cover and refrigerate overnight.
5. In the morning, stir and enjoy cold or warm as desired. Add honey or maple syrup for sweetness if desired.

2. Spinach and Mushroom Egg White Omelette

Ingredients:
- 3 egg whites
- 1/4 cup chopped spinach
- 1/4 cup sliced mushrooms
- 1 tablespoon olive oil
- Salt and pepper, to taste

Instructions:
1. Heat olive oil in a non-stick skillet over medium heat.
2. Add chopped spinach and sliced mushrooms, sautéing until spinach is wilted and mushrooms are tender.

3. Season with salt and pepper to taste.
4. Whisk egg whites in a bowl and pour into the skillet over the vegetables.
5. Cook until the egg whites are set and cooked through.
6. Fold the omelet in half and transfer to a plate.
7. Serve hot with a side of whole grain toast or fresh fruit.

3. Chia Seed Pudding with Mixed Berries

Ingredients:
- 1/4 cup chia seeds
- 1 cup almond milk
- 1 tablespoon honey or maple syrup (optional)
- 1/2 cup mixed berries (blueberries, raspberries, strawberries)

Instructions:
1. In a bowl, mix chia seeds, almond milk, and honey or maple syrup (if using).
2. Stir well and let sit for 10 minutes, then stir again to prevent clumping.
3. Cover and refrigerate for at least 2 hours or overnight until the mixture thickens into a pudding-like consistency.
4. To serve, spoon chia seed pudding into bowls or jars and top with mixed berries.
5. Enjoy chilled for a refreshing and nutrient-packed breakfast.

4. Quinoa Breakfast Bowl with Apples and Cinnamon

Ingredients:
- 1/2 cup cooked quinoa
- 1/2 cup almond milk
- 1 apple, diced
- 1 tablespoon honey or maple syrup
- 1/2 teaspoon ground cinnamon
- Optional toppings: chopped nuts, dried cranberries

Instructions:
1. In a saucepan, heat almond milk over medium heat until warm.
2. Stir in cooked quinoa, diced apple, honey or maple syrup, and ground cinnamon.

3. Cook for 2-3 minutes, stirring occasionally, until the apples are softened and the quinoa is heated through.
4. Remove from heat and transfer to a bowl.
5. Sprinkle with optional toppings like chopped nuts and dried cranberries.
6. Serve warm and enjoy this hearty and satisfying breakfast bowl.

5. Avocado and Smoked Salmon Toast

Ingredients:
- 2 slices whole grain bread, toasted
- 1 ripe avocado
- 2 oz smoked salmon
- 1 tablespoon capers
- Fresh dill, for garnish
- Lemon wedges, for serving

Instructions:
1. Mash the ripe avocado in a bowl and spread it evenly onto the toasted whole grain bread slices.
2. Top each slice with smoked salmon and sprinkle with capers.
3. Garnish with fresh dill.
4. Serve with lemon wedges on the side for added flavor.
5. Enjoy this nutritious and omega-3 rich breakfast toast.

6. Berry Spinach Smoothie

Ingredients:
- 1 cup fresh spinach leaves
- 1/2 cup mixed berries (strawberries, raspberries, blueberries)
- 1/2 banana
- 1/2 cup almond milk
- 1 tablespoon chia seeds
- Optional: honey or maple syrup for sweetness

Instructions:
1. Add spinach leaves, mixed berries, banana, almond milk, and chia seeds to a blender.
2. Blend until smooth and creamy.
3. Taste and add honey or maple syrup for sweetness if desired.
4. Pour into a glass and serve immediately as a refreshing and nutrient-packed smoothie.

7. Mediterranean Breakfast Bowl

Ingredients:
- 1/2 cup cooked quinoa
- 1/4 cup hummus
- 1/4 cup cherry tomatoes, halved
- 1/4 cup cucumber, diced
- 2 tablespoons Kalamata olives, sliced
- 1 tablespoon feta cheese, crumbled
- Fresh parsley, for garnish
- Lemon wedges, for serving

Instructions:
1. In a bowl, layer cooked quinoa with hummus, cherry tomatoes, cucumber, Kalamata olives, and crumbled feta cheese.
2. Garnish with fresh parsley.
3. Serve with lemon wedges on the side for added zest.
4. Enjoy this Mediterranean-inspired breakfast bowl packed with flavor and nutrients.

8. Coconut Yogurt Parfait with Granola

Ingredients:
- 1 cup coconut yogurt
- 1/2 cup granola (choose a low-sugar or homemade option)
- 1/2 cup mixed berries (blueberries, strawberries)
- Optional: drizzle of honey or maple syrup

Instructions:
1. In a serving glass or bowl, layer coconut yogurt with granola and mixed berries.
2. Repeat layers until ingredients are used up.
3. Drizzle with honey or maple syrup for sweetness if desired.
4. Serve immediately and enjoy this creamy, crunchy, and antioxidant-rich parfait.

9. Sweet Potato Hash with Eggs

Ingredients:
- 1 medium sweet potato, peeled and diced
- 1/2 onion, diced
- 1 bell pepper, diced
- 2 tablespoons olive oil
- Salt and pepper, to taste
- 2 eggs
- Fresh parsley, for garnish

Instructions:
1. Heat olive oil in a skillet over medium heat.
2. Add diced sweet potato, onion, and bell pepper to the skillet.
3. Sauté until sweet potatoes are tender and lightly browned, about 10-12 minutes.
4. Season with salt and pepper to taste.
5. Create two wells in the sweet potato mixture and crack one egg into each well.
6. Cover and cook until eggs are set to your liking, about 5-7 minutes.
7. Garnish with fresh parsley and serve hot.

10. Almond Butter Banana Smoothie

Ingredients:
- 1 ripe banana
- 1 tablespoon almond butter
- 1 cup almond milk
- 1 tablespoon honey or maple syrup (optional)
- Ice cubes

Instructions:
1. In a blender, combine ripe banana, almond butter, almond milk, and honey or maple syrup (if using).
2. Add ice cubes for a thicker smoothie consistency.
3. Blend until smooth and creamy.
4. Pour into a glass and serve immediately as a protein-rich and filling breakfast smoothie.

11. Egg and Veggie Muffin Cups

Ingredients:
- 6 eggs
- 1/2 cup diced bell peppers
- 1/2 cup diced spinach
- 1/4 cup diced tomatoes
- Salt and pepper, to taste
- Optional: shredded cheese

Instructions:
1. Preheat the oven to 350°F (175°C). Grease a muffin tin or line with muffin liners.
2. In a bowl, whisk eggs until well combined.
3. Stir in diced bell peppers, spinach, tomatoes, salt, and pepper.
4. Pour egg mixture evenly into each muffin cup, filling about 3/4 full.
5. Optional: sprinkle shredded cheese on top of each muffin cup.
6. Bake for 20-25 minutes, or until eggs are set and lightly golden.
7. Remove from the oven and let cool slightly before serving.

12. Avocado Breakfast Salad

Ingredients:
- 1 avocado, sliced
- 2 cups mixed greens (spinach, arugula)
- 1/2 cup cherry tomatoes, halved
- 1/4 cup cucumber, diced

- 2 hard-boiled eggs, sliced
- Lemon vinaigrette dressing

Instructions:
1. Arrange mixed greens on a plate or bowl.
2. Top with sliced avocado, cherry tomatoes, cucumber, and hard-boiled eggs.
3. Drizzle with lemon vinaigrette dressing.
4. Serve immediately as a refreshing and nutrient-packed breakfast salad.

13. Whole Grain Banana Pancakes

Ingredients:
- 1 cup whole wheat flour
- 1 tablespoon baking powder
- 1/4 teaspoon salt
- 1 ripe banana, mashed
- 1 cup almond milk
- 1 tablespoon honey or maple syrup
- 1 tablespoon coconut oil, melted
- Optional: fresh berries for topping

Instructions:
1. In a bowl, whisk together whole wheat flour, baking powder, and salt.
2. In another bowl, mash ripe banana and stir in almond milk, honey or maple syrup, and melted coconut oil.
3. Pour wet ingredients into dry ingredients and stir until just combined. Do not overmix.
4. Heat a non-stick skillet or griddle over medium heat.
5. Scoop about 1/4 cup of batter onto the skillet for each pancake.
6. Cook for 2-3 minutes, or until bubbles form on the surface of the pancake.
7. Flip and cook for another 1-2 minutes, until golden brown and cooked through.
8. Repeat with remaining batter.
9. Serve warm with fresh berries on top and a drizzle of honey or maple syrup if desired.

14. Greek Yogurt with Honey and Almonds

Ingredients:
- 1 cup Greek yogurt
- 1 tablespoon honey
- 2 tablespoons sliced almonds

Instructions:
1. Spoon Greek yogurt into a bowl.
2. Drizzle honey over the yogurt.
3. Sprinkle with sliced almonds.
4. Serve immediately as a protein-rich and satisfying breakfast option.

15. Veggie and Cheese Breakfast Burrito

Ingredients:
- 1 large whole wheat tortilla
- 2 eggs, scrambled
- 1/4 cup shredded cheddar cheese
- 1/4 cup diced bell peppers
- 1/4 cup diced tomatoes
- Salt and pepper, to taste
- Optional: salsa or avocado for topping

Instructions:
1. Heat a large skillet over medium heat.
2. Add scrambled eggs, shredded cheddar cheese, diced bell peppers, and diced tomatoes to the center of the tortilla.
3. Season with salt and pepper.
4. Fold the sides of the tortilla over the filling to create a burrito.
5. Place the burrito seam-side down on the skillet and cook for 2-3 minutes on each side, until golden brown and cheese is melted.
6. Optional: serve with salsa or avocado on the side for added flavor.

16. Almond Berry Breakfast Quinoa

Ingredients:
- 1/2 cup cooked quinoa
- 1/4 cup almond milk
- 1/2 cup mixed berries (blueberries, raspberries)
- 1 tablespoon almond butter
- Optional: honey or maple syrup for sweetness

Instructions:
1. In a saucepan, heat almond milk over medium heat until warm.
2. Stir in cooked quinoa, mixed berries, and almond butter.
3. Cook for 2-3 minutes, stirring occasionally, until the berries are warmed through.
4. Optional: add honey or maple syrup for sweetness.
5. Serve warm and enjoy this protein-packed breakfast quinoa.

17. Tomato Basil Frittata

Ingredients:
- 4 eggs
- 1/4 cup milk or almond milk
- 1/2 cup cherry tomatoes, halved
- 1/4 cup fresh basil leaves, chopped
- Salt and pepper, to taste
- Optional: shredded mozzarella cheese

Instructions:
1. Preheat the oven to 350°F (175°C).
2. In a bowl, whisk together eggs and milk until well combined.
3. Stir in cherry tomatoes, fresh basil leaves, salt, and pepper.
4. Pour egg mixture into a greased baking dish or skillet.
5. Optional: sprinkle shredded mozzarella cheese on top.
6. Bake for 20-25 minutes, or until eggs are set and lightly golden.

7. Remove from the oven and let cool slightly before slicing and serving.

18. Peanut Butter Banana Smoothie Bowl

Ingredients:
- 1 ripe banana
- 1 tablespoon peanut butter
- 1/2 cup almond milk
- 1/4 cup rolled oats
- Optional toppings: sliced banana, granola, chia seeds

Instructions:
1. In a blender, combine ripe banana, peanut butter, almond milk, and rolled oats.
2. Blend until smooth and creamy.
3. Pour into a bowl and top with optional toppings like sliced banana, granola, and chia seeds.
4. Serve immediately as a filling and nutritious smoothie bowl.

19. Mediterranean Egg Wrap

Ingredients:
- 1 whole wheat wrap or tortilla
- 2 eggs, scrambled
- 1/4 cup diced cucumber
- 1/4 cup cherry tomatoes, halved
- 2 tablespoons crumbled feta cheese
- Fresh parsley, for garnish

Instructions:
1. Heat a large skillet over medium heat.
2. Add scrambled eggs to the center of the wrap or tortilla.
3. Top with diced cucumber, cherry tomatoes, and crumbled feta cheese.
4. Fold the sides of the wrap over the filling to create a wrap.
5. Place the wrap seam-side down on the skillet and cook for 2-3 minutes on each side, until golden brown and heated through.

6. Garnish with fresh parsley and serve warm.

20. Berry Spinach Salad with Poached Eggs

Ingredients:
- 2 cups baby spinach leaves
- 1/2 cup mixed berries (strawberries, blueberries)
- 2 eggs, poached
- 1 tablespoon balsamic vinegar
- 1 tablespoon olive oil
- Salt and pepper, to taste

Instructions:
1. In a bowl, combine baby spinach leaves and mixed berries.
2. In a small saucepan, bring water to a simmer.
3. Crack one egg into a small bowl and gently slide it into the simmering water. Repeat with the second egg.
4. Poach eggs for 3-4 minutes, until whites are set but yolks are still runny.
5. Remove poached eggs with a slotted spoon and place on top of the spinach and berry mixture.
6. Drizzle with balsamic vinegar and olive oil.
7. Season with salt and pepper to taste.
8. Serve immediately as a nutrient-packed and flavorful breakfast salad.

These recipes are designed to be both nutritious and delicious, focusing on ingredients that support brain health and are suitable for individuals managing Alzheimer's disease. Adjust ingredients and portions as needed to fit specific dietary preferences and nutritional requirements. Enjoy creating and sharing these breakfast options in your cookbook!

5. Lunch Recipes

1. Salmon Salad with Lemon-Dill Dressing

Ingredients:
- 4 oz grilled or baked salmon, flaked
- 2 cups mixed greens (spinach, arugula)
- 1/2 cucumber, sliced
- 1/4 cup cherry tomatoes, halved
- 1/4 red onion, thinly sliced
- 1 tablespoon fresh dill, chopped

Lemon-Dill Dressing:
- 2 tablespoons olive oil
- 1 tablespoon fresh lemon juice
- 1 teaspoon Dijon mustard
- 1 teaspoon honey or maple syrup (optional)
- Salt and pepper, to taste

Instructions:
1. In a large bowl, combine mixed greens, cucumber, cherry tomatoes, and red onion.
2. Top with flaked salmon and sprinkle fresh dill over the salad.
3. In a small bowl, whisk together olive oil, lemon juice, Dijon mustard, honey or maple syrup (if using), salt, and pepper.
4. Drizzle dressing over the salad just before serving.
5. Toss gently to combine and enjoy this refreshing and protein-packed salmon salad.

2. Quinoa and Chickpea Buddha Bowl

Ingredients:
- 1/2 cup cooked quinoa
- 1/2 cup chickpeas, rinsed and drained
- 1/2 cup diced cucumber

- 1/2 cup diced bell peppers
- 1/4 cup sliced olives (Kalamata or black)
- 2 tablespoons crumbled feta cheese (optional)

Lemon-Tahini Dressing:
- 2 tablespoons tahini
- 2 tablespoons olive oil
- 1 tablespoon fresh lemon juice
- 1 clove garlic, minced
- Salt and pepper, to taste

Instructions:
1. In a bowl, layer cooked quinoa with chickpeas, cucumber, bell peppers, olives, and crumbled feta cheese (if using).
2. In a small bowl, whisk together tahini, olive oil, lemon juice, garlic, salt, and pepper until smooth.
3. Drizzle dressing over the Buddha bowl just before serving.
4. Toss gently to combine and enjoy this nutrient-dense and flavorful lunch option.

3. Turkey and Avocado Wrap

Ingredients:
- 1 whole wheat wrap or tortilla
- 3 oz sliced turkey breast
- 1/2 avocado, sliced
- 1/4 cup shredded lettuce
- 1/4 cup diced tomatoes
- 1 tablespoon Greek yogurt or hummus (optional)

Instructions:
1. Lay the whole wheat wrap or tortilla on a flat surface.
2. Spread Greek yogurt or hummus (if using) over the wrap.
3. Layer sliced turkey breast, avocado slices, shredded lettuce, and diced tomatoes evenly over the wrap.
4. Roll up tightly to enclose the filling.

5. Slice in half diagonally and serve immediately as a protein-rich and satisfying lunch wrap.

4. Lentil and Vegetable Soup

Ingredients:
- 1 cup dried lentils, rinsed
- 4 cups vegetable broth
- 1 onion, diced
- 2 carrots, diced
- 2 celery stalks, diced
- 2 cloves garlic, minced
- 1 teaspoon dried thyme
- Salt and pepper, to taste
- Fresh parsley, for garnish

Instructions:
1. In a large pot, heat olive oil over medium heat.
2. Add diced onion, carrots, celery, and minced garlic to the pot. Sauté until vegetables are softened, about 5-7 minutes.
3. Stir in dried lentils and dried thyme.
4. Pour in vegetable broth and bring to a boil.
5. Reduce heat to low, cover, and simmer for 20-25 minutes, or until lentils are tender.
6. Season with salt and pepper to taste.
7. Ladle soup into bowls and garnish with fresh parsley.
8. Serve hot and enjoy this hearty and fiber-rich lentil and vegetable soup.

5. Chicken and Vegetable Stir-Fry

Ingredients:
- 1 tablespoon olive oil
- 1 lb boneless, skinless chicken breast, cut into strips
- 1 bell pepper, sliced
- 1 cup broccoli florets

- 1/2 cup snow peas
- 2 tablespoons low-sodium soy sauce
- 1 tablespoon honey or maple syrup
- 1 teaspoon cornstarch (optional, for thickening)
- Cooked brown rice or quinoa, for serving

Instructions:
1. Heat olive oil in a large skillet or wok over medium-high heat.
2. Add chicken strips to the skillet and cook until browned and cooked through, about 5-7 minutes.
3. Add sliced bell pepper, broccoli florets, and snow peas to the skillet. Stir-fry for another 3-4 minutes, until vegetables are tender-crisp.
4. In a small bowl, whisk together soy sauce, honey or maple syrup, and cornstarch (if using).
5. Pour sauce over the chicken and vegetables in the skillet. Stir well to coat evenly and cook for another 1-2 minutes, until sauce is thickened.
6. Remove from heat and serve immediately over cooked brown rice or quinoa.

6. Caprese Salad with Grilled Chicken

Ingredients:
- 4 oz grilled chicken breast, sliced
- 1 cup cherry tomatoes, halved
- 1/2 cup fresh mozzarella balls (bocconcini), halved
- 1/4 cup fresh basil leaves, torn
- 2 tablespoons balsamic glaze
- Salt and pepper, to taste

Instructions:
1. In a large bowl, combine grilled chicken breast slices, cherry tomatoes, fresh mozzarella balls, and torn fresh basil leaves.
2. Drizzle with balsamic glaze.
3. Season with salt and pepper to taste.
4. Toss gently to combine and enjoy this classic and refreshing Caprese salad with grilled chicken.

7. Mediterranean Quinoa Salad

Ingredients:
- 1 cup cooked quinoa
- 1/2 cup cucumber, diced
- 1/2 cup cherry tomatoes, halved
- 1/4 cup Kalamata olives, sliced
- 1/4 cup red onion, thinly sliced
- 1/4 cup crumbled feta cheese
- Fresh parsley, for garnish

Lemon-Olive Oil Dressing:
- 2 tablespoons olive oil
- 1 tablespoon fresh lemon juice
- 1 clove garlic, minced
- Salt and pepper, to taste

Instructions:
1. In a large bowl, combine cooked quinoa with diced cucumber, cherry tomatoes, Kalamata olives, red onion, and crumbled feta cheese.
2. In a small bowl, whisk together olive oil, lemon juice, minced garlic, salt, and pepper until well combined.
3. Drizzle dressing over the quinoa salad just before serving.
4. Toss gently to combine and garnish with fresh parsley.
5. Serve chilled or at room temperature as a flavorful and nutrient-packed Mediterranean-inspired salad.

8. Turkey and Spinach Stuffed Bell Peppers

Ingredients:
- 4 bell peppers, tops removed and seeds removed
- 1 lb ground turkey
- 1 cup cooked quinoa
- 1 cup spinach, chopped
- 1/2 cup shredded mozzarella cheese

- 1/4 cup marinara sauce
- Salt and pepper, to taste

Instructions:
1. Preheat the oven to 375°F (190°C).
2. In a skillet, cook ground turkey over medium heat until browned and cooked through, breaking it into small pieces with a spatula.
3. Stir in cooked quinoa, chopped spinach, shredded mozzarella cheese, marinara sauce, salt, and pepper.
4. Spoon turkey and spinach mixture evenly into each bell pepper.
5. Place stuffed bell peppers upright in a baking dish.
6. Cover with foil and bake for 30 minutes.
7. Remove foil and bake for an additional 10-15 minutes, until bell peppers are tender and filling is heated through.
8. Remove from the oven and let cool slightly before serving.

9. Tuna Salad Stuffed Avocado

Ingredients:
- 2 avocados, halved and pitted
- 1 can (5 oz) tuna, drained
- 1/4 cup diced celery
- 1/4 cup diced red onion
- 1/4 cup diced cucumber
- 2 tablespoons Greek yogurt
- 1 tablespoon lemon juice
- Salt and pepper, to taste

Instructions:
1. In a bowl, combine drained tuna with diced celery, red onion, cucumber, Greek yogurt, lemon juice, salt, and pepper.
2. Mix well until ingredients are evenly combined.
3. Spoon tuna salad mixture into halved and pitted avocados.
4. Serve immediately as a protein-packed and creamy tuna salad stuffed avocado.

10. Pesto Chicken Pasta Salad

Ingredients:
- 8 oz whole wheat pasta, cooked and cooled
- 1 lb grilled or baked chicken breast, diced
- 1 cup cherry tomatoes, halved
- 1/2 cup fresh mozzarella balls (bocconcini), halved
- 1/4 cup sliced black olives
- 1/4 cup pesto sauce (store-bought or homemade)
- Fresh basil leaves, for garnish

Instructions:
1. In a large bowl, combine cooked and cooled whole wheat pasta with diced grilled chicken breast, cherry tomatoes, fresh mozzarella balls, sliced black olives, and pesto sauce.
2. Toss gently until all ingredients are well combined and evenly coated with pesto sauce.
3. Garnish with fresh basil leaves.
4. Serve chilled or at room temperature as a flavorful and satisfying pasta salad option.

11. Spinach and Mushroom Quiche

Ingredients:
- 1 prepared whole wheat pie crust
- 4 eggs
- 1 cup almond milk or milk of choice
- 1 cup fresh spinach, chopped
- 1 cup mushrooms, sliced
- 1/2 cup shredded cheddar cheese
- Salt and pepper, to taste
- Optional: diced onions, bell peppers, or other vegetables

Instructions:
1. Preheat the oven to 375°F (190°C).

2. In a skillet, sauté mushrooms and spinach over medium heat until spinach is wilted and mushrooms are softened.
3. In a bowl, whisk together eggs, almond milk, salt, and pepper until well combined.
4. Stir in sautéed mushrooms, spinach, shredded cheddar cheese, and any optional vegetables.
5. Pour egg mixture into the prepared whole wheat pie crust.
6. Bake for 35-40 minutes, or until quiche is set and lightly golden on top.
7. Remove from the oven and let cool slightly before slicing and serving.

12. Asian Chicken Lettuce Wraps

Ingredients:
- 1 lb ground chicken or turkey
- 1/4 cup hoisin sauce
- 2 tablespoons low-sodium soy sauce
- 1 tablespoon sesame oil
- 2 garlic cloves, minced
- 1 teaspoon fresh ginger, minced
- 1/2 cup shredded carrots
- 1/4 cup chopped green onions
- 1/4 cup chopped fresh cilantro
- Butter lettuce leaves, for wrapping

Instructions:
1. In a skillet, cook ground chicken or turkey over medium heat until browned and cooked through, breaking it into small pieces with a spatula.
2. Stir in hoisin sauce, soy sauce, sesame oil, minced garlic, and minced ginger. Cook for another 2-3 minutes, until flavors are well combined.
3. Remove from heat and stir in shredded carrots, chopped green onions, and fresh cilantro.
4. Spoon chicken mixture into butter lettuce leaves.
5. Serve immediately as flavorful and low-carb lettuce wraps.

13. Veggie and Hummus Sandwich

Ingredients:
- 2 slices whole wheat bread
- 2 tablespoons hummus (store-bought or homemade)
- 1/2 cup mixed greens (spinach, arugula)
- 1/4 cup shredded carrots
- 1/4 cup cucumber slices
- 1/4 avocado, sliced
- Salt and pepper, to taste

Instructions:
1. Spread hummus evenly over one side of each slice of whole wheat bread.
2. Layer mixed greens, shredded carrots, cucumber slices, and sliced avocado on one slice of bread.
3. Season with salt and pepper to taste.
4. Top with the second slice of bread, hummus side down.
5. Slice in half diagonally and serve immediately as a fresh and nutrient-rich veggie and hummus sandwich.

14. Ratatouille

Ingredients:
- 1 eggplant, diced
- 1 zucchini, diced
- 1 yellow squash, diced
- 1 red bell pepper, diced
- 1 onion, diced
- 2 cloves garlic, minced
- 1 can (14 oz) diced tomatoes
- 2 tablespoons olive oil
- 1 teaspoon dried thyme
- Salt and pepper, to taste
- Fresh basil leaves, for garnish

Instructions:
1. In a large pot or Dutch oven, heat olive oil over medium heat.
2. Add diced onion and minced garlic. Sauté until onion is translucent, about 3-4 minutes.
3. Stir in diced eggplant, zucchini, yellow squash, and red bell pepper.
4. Cook for 5-7 minutes, stirring occasionally, until vegetables are slightly softened.
5. Stir in diced tomatoes and dried thyme.
6. Season with salt and pepper to taste.
7. Cover and simmer over low heat for 20-25 minutes, stirring occasionally, until vegetables are tender and flavors are well combined.
8. Remove from heat and garnish with fresh basil leaves before serving.

15. Greek Chicken Pita Wrap

Ingredients:
- 4 small whole wheat pitas, warmed
- 1 lb grilled chicken breast, sliced
- 1/2 cup diced cucumber
- 1/2 cup diced tomatoes
- 1/4 cup sliced red onion
- 1/4 cup crumbled feta cheese
- Greek yogurt or tzatziki sauce, for topping

Instructions:
1. Fill each warmed whole wheat pita with sliced grilled chicken breast.
2. Top with diced cucumber, diced tomatoes, sliced red onion, and crumbled feta cheese.
3. Drizzle with Greek yogurt or tzatziki sauce.
4. Fold the sides of the pita over the filling to create a wrap.
5. Serve immediately as a protein-packed and flavorful Greek chicken pita wrap.

16. Spinach and Berry Salad with Grilled Chicken

Ingredients:
- 4 oz grilled chicken breast, sliced
- 2 cups fresh spinach leaves
- 1/2 cup fresh strawberries, sliced
- 1/4 cup blueberries
- 1/4 cup sliced almonds
- 2 tablespoons crumbled goat cheese (optional)

Balsamic Vinaigrette:
- 2 tablespoons balsamic vinegar
- 1 tablespoon olive oil
- 1 teaspoon honey or maple syrup (optional)
- Salt and pepper, to taste

Instructions:
1. In a large bowl, combine fresh spinach leaves, sliced strawberries, blueberries, sliced almonds, and crumbled goat cheese (if using).
2. Top with sliced grilled chicken breast.
3. In a small bowl, whisk together balsamic vinegar, olive oil, honey or maple syrup (if using), salt, and pepper.
4. Drizzle dressing over the salad just before serving.
5. Toss gently to combine and enjoy this nutrient-rich and flavorful spinach and berry salad.

17. Shrimp and Avocado Salad

Ingredients:
- 8 oz cooked shrimp, peeled and deveined
- 1 avocado, diced
- 1 cup cherry tomatoes, halved
- 1/4 cup red onion, thinly sliced
- 1/4 cup chopped fresh cilantro
- Juice of 1 lime

- Salt and pepper, to taste

Instructions:
1. In a large bowl, combine cooked shrimp, diced avocado, cherry tomatoes, thinly sliced red onion, and chopped fresh cilantro.
2. Squeeze lime juice over the salad.
3. Season with salt and pepper to taste.
4. Toss gently to combine and serve immediately as a light and protein-packed shrimp and avocado salad.

18. Mediterranean Chickpea Salad

Ingredients:
- 1 can (15 oz) chickpeas, rinsed and drained
- 1 cucumber, diced
- 1/2 cup cherry tomatoes, halved
- 1/4 cup diced red onion
- 1/4 cup Kalamata olives, sliced
- 1/4 cup crumbled feta cheese
- Fresh parsley, for garnish

Lemon-Olive Oil Dressing:
- 2 tablespoons olive oil
- 1 tablespoon fresh lemon juice
- 1 clove garlic, minced
- Salt and pepper, to taste

Instructions:
1. In a large bowl, combine chickpeas, diced cucumber, cherry tomatoes, diced red onion, Kalamata olives, and crumbled feta cheese.
2. In a small bowl, whisk together olive oil, lemon juice, minced garlic, salt, and pepper until well combined.
3. Drizzle dressing over the chickpea salad just before serving.
4. Toss gently to combine and garnish with fresh parsley.

5. Serve chilled or at room temperature as a satisfying and Mediterranean-inspired chickpea salad.

19. Turkey and Sweet Potato Hash

Ingredients:
- 1 lb ground turkey
- 2 sweet potatoes, peeled and diced
- 1 bell pepper, diced
- 1/2 onion, diced
- 2 cloves garlic, minced
- 1 teaspoon smoked paprika
- Salt and pepper, to taste
- Fresh parsley, for garnish

Instructions:
1. In a large skillet, cook ground turkey over medium heat until browned and cooked through, breaking it into small pieces with a spatula.
2. Add diced sweet potatoes, diced bell pepper, diced onion, and minced garlic to the skillet.
3. Season with smoked paprika, salt, and pepper to taste.
4. Cook, stirring occasionally, until sweet potatoes are tender and cooked through, about 15-20 minutes.
5. Remove from heat and garnish with fresh parsley before serving.

20. Grilled Vegetable and Quinoa Salad

Ingredients:
- 1 cup cooked quinoa
- 1 zucchini, sliced
- 1 yellow squash, sliced
- 1 red bell pepper, sliced
- 1 red onion, sliced
- 2 tablespoons olive oil
- 2 tablespoons balsamic vinegar

- 1 teaspoon Italian seasoning
- Salt and pepper, to taste

Instructions:
1. Preheat the grill or grill pan over medium-high heat.
2. In a large bowl, toss sliced zucchini, yellow squash, red bell pepper, and red onion with olive oil, balsamic vinegar, Italian seasoning, salt, and pepper until evenly coated.
3. Grill vegetables for 3-4 minutes per side, or until tender and lightly charred.
4. Remove from the grill and let cool slightly.
5. In a large bowl, combine cooked quinoa with grilled vegetables.
6. Toss gently to combine and serve warm or chilled as a flavorful and hearty grilled vegetable and quinoa salad.

6. Dinner Recipes

1. Lemon Garlic Baked Salmon

Ingredients:
- 4 salmon filets
- 2 tablespoons olive oil
- 2 cloves garlic, minced
- Zest and juice of 1 lemon
- Salt and pepper, to taste
- Fresh parsley, for garnish

Instructions:
1. Preheat the oven to 400°F (200°C).
2. Place salmon filets on a baking sheet lined with parchment paper.
3. In a small bowl, whisk together olive oil, minced garlic, lemon zest, lemon juice, salt, and pepper.
4. Brush the mixture over the salmon filets.
5. Bake for 12-15 minutes, or until salmon is cooked through and flakes easily with a fork.
6. Garnish with fresh parsley before serving.
7. Serve warm as a flavorful and heart-healthy lemon garlic baked salmon.

2. Quinoa and Vegetable Stir-Fry

Ingredients:
- 1 cup quinoa, rinsed
- 2 cups water or vegetable broth
- 1 tablespoon olive oil
- 1 onion, diced
- 2 cloves garlic, minced
- 1 bell pepper, diced
- 1 zucchini, diced
- 1 cup broccoli florets
- 1/4 cup low-sodium soy sauce or tamari

- 1 tablespoon sesame oil
- Salt and pepper, to taste
- Sesame seeds, for garnish (optional)

Instructions:
1. In a medium saucepan, bring water or vegetable broth to a boil.
2. Add quinoa, reduce heat to low, cover, and simmer for 15-20 minutes, or until quinoa is cooked and liquid is absorbed.
3. In a large skillet or wok, heat olive oil over medium heat.
4. Add diced onion and minced garlic. Sauté until onion is translucent.
5. Add diced bell pepper, diced zucchini, and broccoli florets to the skillet. Cook until vegetables are tender-crisp.
6. Stir in cooked quinoa, low-sodium soy sauce or tamari, sesame oil, salt, and pepper.
7. Cook for another 2-3 minutes, stirring occasionally, until heated through.
8. Remove from heat and garnish with sesame seeds, if desired.
9. Serve hot as a nutritious and satisfying quinoa and vegetable stir-fry.

3. Mediterranean Chicken Skewers

Ingredients:
- 1 lb chicken breast, cut into cubes
- 1 lemon, juiced and zested
- 2 cloves garlic, minced
- 1 tablespoon olive oil
- 1 teaspoon dried oregano
- Salt and pepper, to taste
- Cherry tomatoes
- Red onion, cut into chunks
- Bell peppers, cut into chunks

Instructions:
1. In a bowl, combine lemon juice and zest, minced garlic, olive oil, dried oregano, salt, and pepper.

2. Add chicken cubes to the bowl and toss to coat evenly. Marinate in the refrigerator for at least 30 minutes.
3. Preheat the grill or grill pan over medium-high heat.
4. Thread marinated chicken cubes onto skewers alternately with cherry tomatoes, red onion chunks, and bell pepper chunks.
5. Grill skewers for 10-12 minutes, turning occasionally, until chicken is cooked through and vegetables are charred.
6. Remove from the grill and let rest for a few minutes.
7. Serve hot as flavorful and protein-packed Mediterranean chicken skewers.

4. Beef and Broccoli Stir-Fry

Ingredients:
- 1 lb flank steak, thinly sliced
- 1/4 cup low-sodium soy sauce
- 2 tablespoons hoisin sauce
- 1 tablespoon cornstarch
- 2 tablespoons olive oil
- 2 cloves garlic, minced
- 1 tablespoon fresh ginger, grated
- 1 head broccoli, cut into florets
- 1 bell pepper, sliced
- Cooked rice, for serving

Instructions:
1. In a bowl, whisk together soy sauce, hoisin sauce, and cornstarch until smooth. Set aside.
2. Heat olive oil in a large skillet or wok over medium-high heat.
3. Add minced garlic and grated ginger. Sauté for 1 minute until fragrant.
4. Add sliced flank steak to the skillet. Stir-fry for 3-4 minutes until browned and cooked through.
5. Add broccoli florets and sliced bell pepper to the skillet. Stir-fry for another 3-4 minutes until vegetables are tender-crisp.
6. Pour the soy sauce mixture over the beef and vegetables. Stir well to coat evenly.
7. Cook for another 1-2 minutes until the sauce thickens.

8. Remove from heat and serve immediately over cooked rice.
9. Enjoy this savory and satisfying beef and broccoli stir-fry.

5. Spinach and Mushroom Stuffed Chicken Breast

Ingredients:
- 4 boneless, skinless chicken breasts
- 1 cup fresh spinach, chopped
- 1 cup mushrooms, sliced
- 1/2 cup shredded mozzarella cheese
- 2 cloves garlic, minced
- 1 tablespoon olive oil
- Salt and pepper, to taste
- Toothpicks or kitchen twine

Instructions:
1. Preheat the oven to 375°F (190°C).
2. In a skillet, heat olive oil over medium heat.
3. Add minced garlic and sauté for 1 minute until fragrant.
4. Add sliced mushrooms to the skillet. Cook for 4-5 minutes until mushrooms are tender.
5. Stir in chopped spinach and cook for another 2-3 minutes until spinach is wilted.
6. Remove skillet from heat and let cool slightly.
7. Make a horizontal slit along the side of each chicken breast to create a pocket.
8. Stuff each chicken breast with the spinach and mushroom mixture and shredded mozzarella cheese.
9. Secure the openings with toothpicks or tie with kitchen twine.
10. Season stuffed chicken breasts with salt and pepper.
11. Place stuffed chicken breasts on a baking sheet lined with parchment paper.
12. Bake for 25-30 minutes, or until chicken is cooked through and juices run clear.
13. Remove from the oven and let rest for a few minutes before serving.
14. Serve hot as a delicious and wholesome spinach and mushroom stuffed chicken breast.

6. Turkey and Vegetable Chili

Ingredients:
- 1 lb ground turkey
- 1 onion, diced
- 2 cloves garlic, minced
- 1 bell pepper, diced
- 1 zucchini, diced
- 1 can (15 oz) kidney beans, drained and rinsed
- 1 can (15 oz) diced tomatoes
- 2 cups low-sodium chicken broth
- 2 tablespoons chili powder
- 1 teaspoon cumin
- Salt and pepper, to taste
- Fresh cilantro, for garnish

Instructions:
1. In a large pot or Dutch oven, cook ground turkey over medium heat until browned and cooked through.
2. Add diced onion and minced garlic to the pot. Sauté for 2-3 minutes until onion is translucent.
3. Add diced bell pepper and diced zucchini. Cook for another 3-4 minutes until vegetables are tender.
4. Stir in kidney beans, diced tomatoes, chicken broth, chili powder, cumin, salt, and pepper.
5. Bring chili to a boil, then reduce heat to low. Simmer uncovered for 20-25 minutes, stirring occasionally.
6. Adjust seasonings to taste.
7. Serve hot, garnished with fresh cilantro, as a hearty and comforting turkey and vegetable chili.

7. Baked Stuffed Peppers with Quinoa and Chickpeas

Ingredients:
- 4 bell peppers, tops removed and seeded

- 1 cup quinoa, cooked
- 1 can (15 oz) chickpeas, drained and rinsed
- 1 cup spinach, chopped
- 1/2 cup feta cheese, crumbled
- 1 tablespoon olive oil
- 2 cloves garlic, minced
- 1 teaspoon dried oregano
- Salt and pepper, to taste

Instructions:
1. Preheat the oven to 375°F (190°C).
2. In a skillet, heat olive oil over medium heat.
3. Add minced garlic and sauté for 1 minute until fragrant.
4. Add chopped spinach to the skillet. Cook for 2-3 minutes until spinach is wilted.
5. In a large bowl, combine cooked quinoa, chickpeas, sautéed spinach with garlic, crumbled feta cheese, dried oregano, salt, and pepper.
6. Stuff each bell pepper with the quinoa and chickpea mixture.
7. Place stuffed peppers upright in a baking dish.
8. Cover the dish with foil and bake for 30-35 minutes, or until peppers are tender.
9. Remove foil and bake for an additional 5 minutes to lightly brown the tops.
10. Remove from the oven and let cool slightly before serving.
11. Serve hot as nutritious and flavorful baked stuffed peppers.

8. Veggie and Tofu Stir-Fry

Ingredients:
- 1 block (14 oz) firm tofu, drained and cubed
- 2 tablespoons soy sauce or tamari
- 1 tablespoon cornstarch
- 1 tablespoon olive oil
- 1 onion, thinly sliced
- 2 bell peppers, thinly sliced
- 1 cup snow peas
- 1 carrot, thinly sliced
- 2 cloves garlic, minced

- 1 tablespoon fresh ginger, grated
- 1/4 cup low-sodium vegetable broth
- Salt and pepper, to taste
- Sesame seeds, for garnish (optional)

Instructions:
1. In a bowl, toss cubed tofu with soy sauce or tamari and cornstarch until evenly coated. Set aside.
2. Heat olive oil in a large skillet or wok over medium-high heat.
3. Add sliced onion and cook for 2-3 minutes until softened.
4. Add sliced bell peppers, snow peas, and sliced carrot to the skillet. Stir-fry for 4-5 minutes until vegetables are tender-crisp.
5. Push vegetables to one side of the skillet. Add minced garlic and grated ginger to the empty side. Sauté for 1 minute until fragrant.
6. Add tofu cubes to the skillet. Cook for 4-5 minutes, stirring gently, until tofu is lightly browned.
7. Stir in low-sodium vegetable broth. Cook for another 1-2 minutes until heated through.
8. Season with salt and pepper to taste.
9. Remove from heat and garnish with sesame seeds, if desired.
10. Serve hot as a nutritious and colorful veggie and tofu stir-fry.

9. Lemon Herb Chicken with Roasted Vegetables

Ingredients:
- 4 chicken breasts, boneless and skinless
- 2 tablespoons olive oil
- Zest and juice of 1 lemon
- 2 cloves garlic, minced
- 1 tablespoon fresh thyme leaves
- 1 tablespoon fresh rosemary, chopped
- Salt and pepper, to taste
- 2 cups mixed vegetables (such as carrots, potatoes, Brussels sprouts), chopped

Instructions:

1. Preheat the oven to 400°F (200°C).
2. In a bowl, whisk together olive oil, lemon zest, lemon juice, minced garlic, fresh thyme leaves, fresh rosemary, salt, and pepper.
3. Place chicken breasts and mixed vegetables on a baking sheet lined with parchment paper.
4. Brush the lemon herb mixture over the chicken breasts and vegetables.
5. Bake for 25-30 minutes, or until chicken is cooked through and vegetables are tender.
6. Remove from the oven and let rest for a few minutes before serving.
7. Serve hot as a delicious and aromatic lemon herb chicken with roasted vegetables.

10. Lentil and Vegetable Curry

Ingredients:
- 1 cup dried lentils, rinsed
- 2 cups vegetable broth
- 1 tablespoon olive oil
- 1 onion, diced
- 2 cloves garlic, minced
- 1 tablespoon curry powder
- 1 teaspoon ground turmeric
- 1 can (15 oz) coconut milk
- 2 cups mixed vegetables (such as cauliflower, bell peppers, peas)
- Salt and pepper, to taste
- Fresh cilantro, for garnish

Instructions:
1. In a medium saucepan, combine dried lentils and vegetable broth. Bring to a boil, then reduce heat to low. Simmer, covered, for 15-20 minutes, or until lentils are tender.
2. In a large skillet or pot, heat olive oil over medium heat.
3. Add diced onion and minced garlic. Sauté for 2-3 minutes until onion is translucent.
4. Stir in curry powder and ground turmeric. Cook for 1 minute until fragrant.

5. Add coconut milk and mixed vegetables to the skillet. Bring to a simmer and cook for 10-12 minutes, or until vegetables are tender.
6. Stir in cooked lentils. Season with salt and pepper to taste.
7. Cook for another 2-3 minutes until heated through.
8. Remove from heat and garnish with fresh cilantro.
9. Serve hot with rice or naan as a flavorful and satisfying lentil and vegetable curry.

11. Herb-Crusted Baked Chicken Thighs

Ingredients:
- 4 chicken thighs, bone-in and skin-on
- 2 tablespoons olive oil
- 1 tablespoon Dijon mustard
- 1 tablespoon fresh thyme leaves, chopped
- 1 tablespoon fresh rosemary, chopped
- 2 cloves garlic, minced
- Salt and pepper, to taste

Instructions:
1. Preheat the oven to 400°F (200°C).
2. In a small bowl, whisk together olive oil, Dijon mustard, chopped thyme leaves, chopped rosemary, minced garlic, salt, and pepper.
3. Place chicken thighs on a baking sheet lined with parchment paper.
4. Brush the herb mixture over the chicken thighs, coating evenly.
5. Bake for 30-35 minutes, or until chicken is golden brown and cooked through.
6. Remove from the oven and let rest for a few minutes before serving.
7. Serve hot as flavorful and herb-crusted baked chicken thighs.

12. Mediterranean Quinoa Salad with Grilled Chicken

Ingredients:
- 1 cup quinoa, rinsed
- 2 cups water or vegetable broth
- 2 chicken breasts, boneless and skinless

- 1 tablespoon olive oil
- 1 teaspoon dried oregano
- Salt and pepper, to taste
- 1 cucumber, diced
- 1 cup cherry tomatoes, halved
- 1/2 cup Kalamata olives, pitted and sliced
- 1/4 cup red onion, thinly sliced
- 1/4 cup crumbled feta cheese
- Fresh parsley, for garnish

Instructions:
1. In a medium saucepan, bring water or vegetable broth to a boil.
2. Add quinoa, reduce heat to low, cover, and simmer for 15-20 minutes, or until quinoa is cooked and liquid is absorbed.
3. Preheat the grill or grill pan over medium-high heat.
4. Rub chicken breasts with olive oil, dried oregano, salt, and pepper.
5. Grill chicken breasts for 6-7 minutes per side, or until cooked through and no longer pink in the center.
6. Remove chicken from the grill and let rest for a few minutes before slicing.
7. In a large bowl, combine cooked quinoa, diced cucumber, halved cherry tomatoes, sliced Kalamata olives, thinly sliced red onion, and crumbled feta cheese.
8. Toss salad ingredients together.
9. Arrange sliced grilled chicken on top of the quinoa salad.
10. Garnish with fresh parsley before serving.
11. Serve chilled or at room temperature as a refreshing and protein-packed Mediterranean quinoa salad with grilled chicken.

13. Cauliflower Fried Rice with Shrimp

Ingredients:
- 1 head cauliflower, grated (or 4 cups cauliflower rice)
- 1 lb shrimp, peeled and deveined
- 2 tablespoons olive oil
- 2 cloves garlic, minced

- 1 tablespoon fresh ginger, grated
- 1 cup mixed vegetables (such as peas, carrots, bell peppers)
- 2 tablespoons low-sodium soy sauce or tamari
- 1 tablespoon sesame oil
- 2 eggs, beaten (optional)
- Salt and pepper, to taste
- Green onions, sliced, for garnish

Instructions:
1. In a large skillet or wok, heat olive oil over medium heat.
2. Add minced garlic and grated ginger. Sauté for 1 minute until fragrant.
3. Add shrimp to the skillet. Cook for 2-3 minutes until shrimp turn pink and opaque. Remove shrimp from skillet and set aside.
4. In the same skillet, add mixed vegetables. Stir-fry for 3-4 minutes until vegetables are tender-crisp.
5. Push vegetables to one side of the skillet. Pour beaten eggs into the empty side. Scramble eggs until cooked through.
6. Stir in grated cauliflower (cauliflower rice) to the skillet.
7. Add low-sodium soy sauce or tamari and sesame oil. Stir well to combine.
8. Return cooked shrimp to the skillet. Mix everything together.
9. Cook for another 2-3 minutes until heated through.
10. Season with salt and pepper to taste.
11. Remove from heat and garnish with sliced green onions.
12. Serve hot as a nutritious and low-carb cauliflower fried rice with shrimp.

14. Sweet Potato and Black Bean Enchiladas

Ingredients:
- 2 large sweet potatoes, peeled and diced
- 1 can (15 oz) black beans, drained and rinsed
- 1 tablespoon olive oil
- 1 onion, diced
- 2 cloves garlic, minced
- 1 teaspoon ground cumin
- 1 teaspoon chili powder

- Salt and pepper, to taste
- 8 whole wheat or corn tortillas
- 1 can (15 oz) enchilada sauce
- 1 cup shredded cheddar cheese
- Fresh cilantro, for garnish

Instructions:
1. Preheat the oven to 375°F (190°C).
2. Place diced sweet potatoes in a microwave-safe bowl. Cover with a damp paper towel and microwave for 4-5 minutes, or until tender.
3. In a large skillet, heat olive oil over medium heat.
4. Add diced onion and minced garlic. Sauté for 2-3 minutes until onion is translucent.
5. Stir in cooked sweet potatoes, black beans, ground cumin, chili powder, salt, and pepper. Cook for 2-3 minutes until heated through.
6. Spread a small amount of enchilada sauce on the bottom of a baking dish.
7. Fill each tortilla with the sweet potato and black bean mixture. Roll up and place seam-side down in the baking dish.
8. Pour remaining enchilada sauce over the rolled tortillas.
9. Sprinkle shredded cheddar cheese evenly over the top.
10. Bake for 20-25 minutes, or until the cheese is melted and bubbly.
11. Remove from the oven and let cool slightly before serving.
12. Garnish with fresh cilantro.
13. Serve hot as delicious and satisfying sweet potato and black bean enchiladas.

15. Salmon with Asparagus and Lemon Butter Sauce

Ingredients:
- 4 salmon filets
- 1 lb asparagus, trimmed
- 2 tablespoons olive oil
- 2 tablespoons butter
- Zest and juice of 1 lemon
- 2 cloves garlic, minced
- Salt and pepper, to taste

- Fresh dill, for garnish

Instructions:
1. Preheat the oven to 400°F (200°C).
2. Place asparagus on a baking sheet lined with parchment paper. Drizzle with olive oil, salt, and pepper. Toss to coat.
3. Place salmon filets on the baking sheet with the asparagus.
4. In a small saucepan, melt butter over medium heat.
5. Add minced garlic and sauté for 1 minute until fragrant.
6. Remove the saucepan from heat. Stir in lemon zest and juice.
7. Brush the lemon butter sauce over the salmon filets.
8. Bake for 12-15 minutes, or until salmon is cooked through and flakes easily with a fork.
9. Roast asparagus in the oven for 10-12 minutes, or until tender.
10. Remove from the oven and let rest for a few minutes before serving.
11. Garnish salmon with fresh dill before serving.
12. Serve hot as a delightful and nutritious salmon with asparagus and lemon butter sauce.

16. Roasted Vegetable Quinoa Bowls

Ingredients:
- 1 cup quinoa, rinsed
- 2 cups water or vegetable broth
- 1 sweet potato, peeled and diced
- 1 zucchini, diced
- 1 bell pepper, diced
- 1 red onion, thinly sliced
- 2 tablespoons olive oil
- 1 teaspoon dried thyme
- Salt and pepper, to taste
- 1/4 cup crumbled feta cheese or goat cheese (optional)
- Fresh parsley, for garnish

Instructions:
1. Preheat the oven to 400°F (200°C).
2. In a medium saucepan, bring water or vegetable broth to a boil.
3. Add quinoa, reduce heat to low, cover, and simmer for 15-20 minutes, or until quinoa is cooked and liquid is absorbed.
4. Meanwhile, spread diced sweet potato, diced zucchini, diced bell pepper, and thinly sliced red onion on a baking sheet lined with parchment paper.
5. Drizzle olive oil over the vegetables. Sprinkle with dried thyme, salt, and pepper. Toss to coat evenly.
6. Roast vegetables in the preheated oven for 20-25 minutes, stirring halfway through, until vegetables are tender and slightly caramelized.
7. Fluff cooked quinoa with a fork and divided among serving bowls.
8. Top quinoa with roasted vegetables.
9. If desired, sprinkle crumbled feta cheese or goat cheese over the bowls.
10. Garnish with fresh parsley before serving.
11. Serve warm as nutritious and flavorful roasted vegetable quinoa bowls.

17. Beef and Broccoli Stir-Fry

Ingredients:
- 1 lb flank steak, thinly sliced
- 1/4 cup low-sodium soy sauce or tamari
- 2 tablespoons oyster sauce
- 2 tablespoons rice vinegar
- 1 tablespoon cornstarch
- 1 tablespoon sesame oil
- 2 tablespoons olive oil
- 2 cloves garlic, minced
- 1 tablespoon fresh ginger, grated
- 1 head broccoli, cut into florets
- 1 bell pepper, thinly sliced
- 1/2 cup low-sodium beef broth
- Salt and pepper, to taste
- Sesame seeds, for garnish (optional)
- Green onions, sliced, for garnish (optional)

Instructions:
1. In a bowl, whisk together soy sauce or tamari, oyster sauce, rice vinegar, cornstarch, and sesame oil.
2. Add thinly sliced flank steak to the bowl. Toss to coat the steak in the marinade. Set aside for 10-15 minutes.
3. In a large skillet or wok, heat olive oil over medium-high heat.
4. Add minced garlic and grated ginger. Sauté for 1 minute until fragrant.
5. Add marinated flank steak to the skillet in a single layer. Cook for 2-3 minutes per side until browned and cooked through. Remove steak from skillet and set aside.
6. In the same skillet, add broccoli florets and thinly sliced bell pepper. Stir-fry for 4-5 minutes until vegetables are tender-crisp.
7. Return cooked steak to the skillet. Pour in low-sodium beef broth. Stir well to combine and heat through.
8. Season with salt and pepper to taste.
9. Remove from heat and garnish with sesame seeds and sliced green onions, if desired.
10. Serve hot as a savory and satisfying beef and broccoli stir-fry.

18. Quinoa Stuffed Bell Peppers

Ingredients:
- 4 bell peppers, tops removed and seeded
- 1 cup quinoa, rinsed
- 2 cups water or vegetable broth
- 1 can (15 oz) black beans, drained and rinsed
- 1 cup corn kernels (fresh or frozen)
- 1 cup cherry tomatoes, halved
- 1/2 cup shredded cheddar cheese
- 1 tablespoon olive oil
- 1 teaspoon ground cumin
- 1 teaspoon chili powder
- Salt and pepper, to taste
- Fresh cilantro, for garnish

Instructions:
1. Preheat the oven to 375°F (190°C).
2. In a medium saucepan, bring water or vegetable broth to a boil.
3. Add quinoa, reduce heat to low, cover, and simmer for 15-20 minutes, or until quinoa is cooked and liquid is absorbed.
4. In a large bowl, combine cooked quinoa, black beans, corn kernels, halved cherry tomatoes, shredded cheddar cheese, olive oil, ground cumin, chili powder, salt, and pepper.
5. Stuff each bell pepper with the quinoa mixture, pressing lightly to pack.
6. Place stuffed peppers upright in a baking dish.
7. Cover the dish with foil and bake for 30-35 minutes, or until peppers are tender.
8. Remove foil and sprinkle additional shredded cheddar cheese on top, if desired.
9. Bake uncovered for another 5 minutes until the cheese is melted and bubbly.
10. Remove from the oven and let cool slightly before serving.
11. Garnish with fresh cilantro before serving.
12. Serve hot as delicious and wholesome quinoa stuffed bell peppers.

19. Chicken and Vegetable Sheet Pan Dinner

Ingredients:
- 4 chicken thighs, bone-in and skin-on
- 1 lb baby potatoes, halved
- 1 bunch asparagus, trimmed
- 1 pint cherry tomatoes
- 2 tablespoons olive oil
- 2 cloves garlic, minced
- 1 tablespoon fresh rosemary, chopped
- 1 tablespoon fresh thyme leaves
- Salt and pepper, to taste
- Lemon wedges, for serving (optional)

Instructions:
1. Preheat the oven to 400°F (200°C).
2. Place chicken thighs, halved baby potatoes, trimmed asparagus, and cherry tomatoes on a large baking sheet.

3. Drizzle olive oil over the ingredients on the baking sheet.
4. Sprinkle minced garlic, chopped fresh rosemary, chopped fresh thyme leaves, salt, and pepper evenly over everything.
5. Toss to coat all ingredients in the olive oil and seasonings.
6. Arrange chicken thighs skin-side up and evenly spaced on the baking sheet.
7. Roast in the preheated oven for 35-40 minutes, or until chicken is cooked through and potatoes are tender.
8. Remove from the oven and let rest for a few minutes before serving.
9. Serve hot with lemon wedges on the side, if desired.
10. Enjoy this easy and flavorful chicken and vegetable sheet pan dinner.

20. Spinach and Mushroom Stuffed Chicken Breast

Ingredients:
- 4 boneless, skinless chicken breasts
- 2 cups fresh spinach leaves
- 1 cup mushrooms, sliced
- 1/2 cup shredded mozzarella cheese
- 2 tablespoons olive oil
- 2 cloves garlic, minced
- Salt and pepper, to taste
- Toothpicks or kitchen twine

Instructions:
1. Preheat the oven to 375°F (190°C).
2. In a skillet, heat olive oil over medium heat.
3. Add minced garlic and sauté for 1 minute until fragrant.
4. Add sliced mushrooms to the skillet. Cook for 5-6 minutes until mushrooms are softened and lightly browned.
5. Add fresh spinach leaves to the skillet. Cook for 1-2 minutes until spinach is wilted. Remove skillet from heat and let cool slightly.
6. Butterfly each chicken breast by slicing horizontally almost all the way through, so it opens like a book.
7. Season the inside of each chicken breast with salt and pepper.
8. Spoon the mushroom and spinach mixture evenly onto each chicken breast.

9. Sprinkle shredded mozzarella cheese over the spinach and mushroom mixture.

10. Fold the chicken breast over the filling and secure with toothpicks or tie with kitchen twine.

11. Place stuffed chicken breasts on a baking sheet lined with parchment paper.

12. Bake in the preheated oven for 25-30 minutes, or until chicken is cooked through and juices run clear.

13. Remove from the oven and let rest for a few minutes before serving.

14. Serve hot as delicious and nutritious spinach and mushroom stuffed chicken breast.

7. Snacks and Appetizers

1. Greek Yogurt with Berries and Almonds

Ingredients:
- 1 cup Greek yogurt
- 1/2 cup mixed berries (such as strawberries, blueberries, raspberries)
- 2 tablespoons sliced almonds
- Optional: drizzle of honey or maple syrup

Instructions:
1. Spoon Greek yogurt into a serving bowl.
2. Top with mixed berries and sliced almonds.
3. Drizzle with honey or maple syrup if desired.
4. Serve immediately as a refreshing and protein-packed snack.

2. Avocado and Tomato Bruschetta

Ingredients:
- 1 ripe avocado, mashed
- 1 cup cherry tomatoes, diced
- 1 clove garlic, minced
- 1 tablespoon fresh basil, chopped
- 1 tablespoon balsamic vinegar
- Salt and pepper, to taste
- Whole grain baguette, sliced and toasted

Instructions:
1. In a bowl, combine mashed avocado, diced cherry tomatoes, minced garlic, chopped fresh basil, balsamic vinegar, salt, and pepper.
2. Spread avocado mixture onto toasted whole grain baguette slices.
3. Serve immediately as a flavorful and nutrient-rich bruschetta.

3. Apple Slices with Almond Butter

Ingredients:
- 1 apple, cored and sliced
- 2 tablespoons almond butter
- Optional: sprinkle of cinnamon

Instructions:
1. Arrange apple slices on a plate.
2. Serve with almond butter for dipping.
3. Optional: sprinkle cinnamon over apple slices before serving.
4. Enjoy this simple and satisfying snack option.

4. Hummus with Raw Vegetables

Ingredients:
- 1 cup hummus (store-bought or homemade)
- Assorted raw vegetables (carrot sticks, cucumber slices, bell pepper strips, cherry tomatoes)

Instructions:
1. Place hummus in a serving bowl.
2. Arrange raw vegetables around the hummus bowl.
3. Serve immediately as a nutritious and crunchy snack.

5. Trail Mix

Ingredients:
- 1 cup mixed nuts (almonds, walnuts, cashews)
- 1/2 cup dried fruit (raisins, cranberries)
- 1/4 cup dark chocolate chips or chunks

Instructions:
1. In a bowl, combine mixed nuts, dried fruit, and dark chocolate chips.
2. Toss gently to mix.

3. Serve in individual portions as a convenient and energizing snack.

6. Caprese Skewers

Ingredients:
- Cherry tomatoes
- Fresh mozzarella balls
- Fresh basil leaves
- Balsamic glaze or reduction

Instructions:
1. Thread cherry tomatoes, fresh mozzarella balls, and fresh basil leaves onto skewers.
2. Arrange skewers on a serving platter.
3. Drizzle with balsamic glaze or reduction just before serving.
4. Serve as a colorful and elegant appetizer option.

7. Cucumber Bites with Herbed Cream Cheese

Ingredients:
- 1 cucumber, sliced into rounds
- 4 oz cream cheese, softened
- 1 tablespoon fresh dill, chopped
- 1 tablespoon fresh chives, chopped
- Salt and pepper, to taste

Instructions:
1. In a bowl, mix softened cream cheese with chopped fresh dill, chopped fresh chives, salt, and pepper until well combined.
2. Spread herbed cream cheese on cucumber rounds.
3. Serve immediately as a refreshing and creamy appetizer.

8. Stuffed Mini Bell Peppers

Ingredients:
- Mini bell peppers
- 4 oz goat cheese, softened
- 1/4 cup chopped fresh parsley
- 1/4 cup chopped walnuts
- Optional: drizzle of honey

Instructions:
1. Preheat the oven to 375°F (190°C).
2. Cut mini bell peppers in half lengthwise and remove seeds.
3. In a bowl, mix softened goat cheese with chopped fresh parsley and chopped walnuts.
4. Spoon goat cheese mixture into each mini bell pepper half.
5. Optional: drizzle honey over stuffed peppers.
6. Bake for 10-12 minutes, or until peppers are tender and goat cheese is lightly browned.
7. Serve warm as a flavorful and savory appetizer.

9. Smoked Salmon Cucumber Bites

Ingredients:
- English cucumber, sliced into rounds
- Smoked salmon slices
- 4 oz cream cheese, softened
- Fresh dill, for garnish

Instructions:
1. Spread softened cream cheese on cucumber rounds.
2. Top each cucumber round with a slice of smoked salmon.
3. Garnish with fresh dill.
4. Serve immediately as an elegant and protein-rich appetizer.

10. Mediterranean Hummus Platter

Ingredients:
- 1 cup hummus (store-bought or homemade)
- Cherry tomatoes
- Cucumber slices
- Kalamata olives
- Feta cheese, cubed
- Pita bread or whole grain crackers

Instructions:
1. Spread hummus onto a serving platter.
2. Arrange cherry tomatoes, cucumber slices, Kalamata olives, and cubed feta cheese around the hummus.
3. Serve with pita bread or whole grain crackers.
4. Enjoy this Mediterranean-inspired appetizer platter.

11. Cottage Cheese with Fresh Fruit

Ingredients:
- 1 cup low-fat cottage cheese
- 1/2 cup mixed fresh fruit (such as berries, kiwi, mango)

Instructions:
1. Spoon cottage cheese into a serving bowl.
2. Top with mixed fresh fruit.
3. Serve immediately as a protein-packed and refreshing snack.

12. Almond Butter Energy Balls

Ingredients:
- 1 cup rolled oats
- 1/2 cup almond butter
- 1/4 cup honey or maple syrup
- 1/4 cup ground flaxseed

- 1/4 cup mini dark chocolate chips
- 1 teaspoon vanilla extract

Instructions:
1. In a bowl, mix together rolled oats, almond butter, honey or maple syrup, ground flaxseed, mini dark chocolate chips, and vanilla extract until well combined.
2. Roll mixture into small balls using your hands.
3. Place energy balls on a baking sheet lined with parchment paper.
4. Chill in the refrigerator for at least 30 minutes before serving.
5. Enjoy these nutritious and energizing almond butter energy balls as a convenient snack option.

13. Greek Yogurt Parfait

Ingredients:
- 1 cup Greek yogurt
- 1/2 cup granola (low-sugar or homemade)
- 1/2 cup mixed fresh berries (such as strawberries, blueberries)

Instructions:
1. In a serving glass or bowl, layer Greek yogurt, granola, and mixed fresh berries.
2. Repeat layers as desired.
3. Serve immediately as a creamy, crunchy, and fruity Greek yogurt parfait.

14. Edamame with Sea Salt

Ingredients:
- 1 cup edamame (shelled)
- Sea salt, to taste

Instructions:
1. Steam or boil edamame according to package instructions until tender.
2. Drain and transfer edamame to a serving bowl.
3. Sprinkle it with sea salt to taste.
4. Serve warm or chilled as a protein-rich and satisfying snack.

15. Baked Kale Chips

Ingredients:
- 1 bunch kale, washed and dried
- 1 tablespoon olive oil
- Salt, to taste

Instructions:
1. Preheat the oven to 300°F (150°C).
2. Remove kale leaves from stems and tear into bite-sized pieces.
3. In a bowl, toss kale pieces with olive oil until evenly coated.
4. Arrange kale pieces in a single layer on a baking sheet lined with parchment paper.
5. Sprinkle it with salt to taste.
6. Bake for 10-15 minutes, or until kale chips are crispy.
7. Remove from the oven and let cool before serving.
8. Enjoy these crunchy and nutritious baked kale chips as a guilt-free snack.

16. Tomato Basil Bruschetta

Ingredients:
- 1 baguette, sliced and toasted
- 2 cups cherry tomatoes, diced
- 1/4 cup fresh basil leaves, chopped
- 2 tablespoons balsamic vinegar
- 1 tablespoon olive oil
- 1 clove garlic, minced
- Salt and pepper, to taste

Instructions:
1. In a bowl, combine diced cherry tomatoes, chopped fresh basil leaves, balsamic vinegar, olive oil, minced garlic, salt, and pepper.
2. Spoon tomato basil mixture onto toasted baguette slices.
3. Serve immediately as a classic and flavorful tomato basil bruschetta.

17. Cucumber Rolls with Herbed Cream Cheese and Smoked Salmon

Ingredients:
- 1 English cucumber
- 4 oz cream cheese, softened
- 1 tablespoon fresh dill, chopped
- 1 tablespoon fresh chives, chopped
- 4 oz smoked salmon slices

Instructions:
1. Using a vegetable peeler, peel long strips from the cucumber lengthwise.
2. In a bowl, mix softened cream cheese with chopped fresh dill and chopped fresh chives until well combined.
3. Spread herbed cream cheese onto cucumber strips.
4. Top each cucumber strip with smoked salmon slices.
5. Roll up cucumber strips and secure with toothpicks if needed.
6. Serve immediately as an elegant and savory appetizer.

18. Stuffed Mushrooms with Spinach and Feta

Ingredients:
- 12 large mushrooms, stems removed
- 1 tablespoon olive oil
- 1 cup fresh spinach, chopped
- 1/2 cup crumbled feta cheese
- 2 cloves garlic, minced
- Salt and pepper, to taste

Instructions:
1. Preheat the oven to 375°F (190°C).
2. In a skillet, heat olive oil over medium heat.
3. Add chopped fresh spinach and minced garlic. Sauté until spinach is wilted.
4. Remove skillet from heat and stir in crumbled feta cheese, salt, and pepper.
5. Spoon spinach and feta mixture into mushroom caps.
6. Place stuffed mushrooms on a baking sheet lined with parchment paper.

7. Bake for 15-20 minutes, or until mushrooms are tender and filling is lightly browned.
8. Serve warm as a flavorful and satisfying appetizer.

19. Mediterranean Cucumber Cups

Ingredients:
- 2 large cucumbers
- 1 cup cherry tomatoes, halved
- 1/2 cup Kalamata olives, sliced
- 1/4 cup crumbled feta cheese
- Fresh parsley, for garnish
- Lemon juice, for drizzling

Instructions:
1. Slice cucumbers into thick rounds.
2. Use a melon baller or spoon to hollow out centers of cucumber rounds, creating cups.
3. In a bowl, combine cherry tomatoes, sliced Kalamata olives, and crumbled feta cheese.
4. Spoon tomato and olive mixture into cucumber cups.
5. Garnish with fresh parsley and drizzle with lemon juice.
6. Serve immediately as a refreshing and Mediterranean-inspired appetizer.

20. Smoked Salmon and Avocado Crostini

Ingredients:
- Baguette, sliced and toasted
- 4 oz cream cheese, softened
- 4 oz smoked salmon slices
- 1 avocado, sliced
- Fresh dill, for garnish

Instructions:
1. Spread softened cream cheese on toasted baguette slices.

2. Top each baguette slice with smoked salmon slices and sliced avocado.
3. Garnish with fresh dill.
4. Serve immediately as an elegant and delicious smoked salmon and avocado crostini.

8. Desserts

1. Berry Yogurt Parfait

Ingredients:
- 1 cup Greek yogurt (plain or vanilla, low-fat)
- 1 cup mixed berries (such as strawberries, blueberries, raspberries)
- 1/4 cup granola (low-sugar, optional)
- 1 tablespoon honey (optional)
- Fresh mint leaves, for garnish

Instructions:
1. In a serving glass or bowl, layer Greek yogurt, mixed berries, and granola (if using).
2. Drizzle with honey for added sweetness, if desired.
3. Garnish with fresh mint leaves.
4. Serve chilled as a refreshing and nutritious berry yogurt parfait.

2. Baked Apples with Cinnamon and Walnuts

Ingredients:
- 4 apples (such as Granny Smith or Honeycrisp), cored
- 1/4 cup chopped walnuts
- 1 tablespoon honey or maple syrup
- 1 teaspoon ground cinnamon
- 1/4 cup water

Instructions:
1. Preheat the oven to 375°F (190°C).
2. In a small bowl, combine chopped walnuts, honey or maple syrup, and ground cinnamon.
3. Stuff each cored apple with the walnut mixture.
4. Place stuffed apples in a baking dish.
5. Pour water into the baking dish around the apples.
6. Cover with foil and bake for 25-30 minutes, or until the apples are tender.

7. Remove foil and bake for an additional 5 minutes to slightly caramelize the tops.
8. Remove from the oven and let cool slightly before serving.
9. Serve warm as comforting and aromatic baked apples with cinnamon and walnuts.

3. Chia Seed Pudding with Berries

Ingredients:
- 1/4 cup chia seeds
- 1 cup almond milk or coconut milk (unsweetened)
- 1 tablespoon honey or maple syrup (optional)
- 1/2 teaspoon vanilla extract
- 1 cup mixed berries (such as strawberries, blueberries, raspberries)
- Fresh mint leaves, for garnish

Instructions:
1. In a mixing bowl, combine chia seeds, almond milk or coconut milk, honey or maple syrup (if using), and vanilla extract.
2. Stir well to combine.
3. Cover and refrigerate for at least 2 hours or overnight, until the mixture thickens to a pudding-like consistency.
4. Stir the chia seed pudding before serving to ensure even texture.
5. Spoon chia seed pudding into serving bowls or glasses.
6. Top with mixed berries.
7. Garnish with fresh mint leaves.
8. Serve chilled as a nutritious and filling chia seed pudding with berries.

4. Banana Oatmeal Cookies

Ingredients:
- 2 ripe bananas, mashed
- 1 cup old-fashioned oats
- 1/4 cup chopped nuts (such as walnuts or almonds)
- 1/4 cup dried fruit (such as raisins or cranberries)
- 1 teaspoon ground cinnamon

- 1/4 teaspoon salt
- 1/4 cup dark chocolate chips (optional)

Instructions:
1. Preheat the oven to 350°F (175°C). Line a baking sheet with parchment paper.
2. In a mixing bowl, combine mashed bananas, old-fashioned oats, chopped nuts, dried fruit, ground cinnamon, salt, and dark chocolate chips (if using).
3. Stir well until all ingredients are fully incorporated.
4. Drop spoonfuls of the cookie dough onto the prepared baking sheet, spacing them apart.
5. Flatten each cookie slightly with the back of a spoon or your fingers.
6. Bake for 15-18 minutes, or until cookies are golden brown and set.
7. Remove from the oven and let cool on the baking sheet for 5 minutes.
8. Transfer cookies to a wire rack to cool completely.
9. Serve as wholesome and naturally sweet banana oatmeal cookies.

5. Mixed Berry Sorbet

Ingredients:
- 2 cups mixed berries (such as strawberries, blueberries, raspberries)
- 1/4 cup honey or maple syrup
- 1 tablespoon lemon juice
- Fresh mint leaves, for garnish

Instructions:
1. In a blender or food processor, combine mixed berries, honey or maple syrup, and lemon juice.
2. Blend until smooth and well combined.
3. Pour the berry mixture into a shallow dish or baking pan.
4. Cover with plastic wrap and freeze for 3-4 hours, or until firm.
5. Remove from the freezer and let sit at room temperature for 5-10 minutes to slightly soften.
6. Scoop sorbet into serving bowls.
7. Garnish with fresh mint leaves.
8. Serve immediately as refreshing and naturally sweet mixed berry sorbet.

6. Avocado Chocolate Mousse

Ingredients:
- 2 ripe avocados, peeled and pitted
- 1/4 cup unsweetened cocoa powder
- 1/4 cup honey or maple syrup
- 1 teaspoon vanilla extract
- Pinch of salt
- Fresh berries, for garnish

Instructions:
1. In a food processor or blender, combine ripe avocados, unsweetened cocoa powder, honey or maple syrup, vanilla extract, and a pinch of salt.
2. Blend until smooth and creamy, scraping down the sides as needed.
3. Taste and adjust sweetness if desired by adding more honey or maple syrup.
4. Spoon avocado chocolate mousse into serving bowls or glasses.
5. Cover and refrigerate for at least 30 minutes to chill.
6. Garnish with fresh berries before serving.
7. Serve chilled as a decadent and creamy avocado chocolate mousse.

7. Coconut Macaroons

Ingredients:
- 2 cups unsweetened shredded coconut
- 1/2 cup coconut flour
- 1/2 cup coconut oil, melted
- 1/2 cup honey or maple syrup
- 1 teaspoon vanilla extract
- Pinch of salt
- Dark chocolate, melted (optional, for drizzling)

Instructions:
1. Preheat the oven to 350°F (175°C). Line a baking sheet with parchment paper.
2. In a mixing bowl, combine unsweetened shredded coconut, coconut flour, melted coconut oil, honey or maple syrup, vanilla extract, and a pinch of salt.

3. Stir well until all ingredients are fully incorporated and the mixture holds together.
4. Scoop tablespoon-sized portions of the mixture and shape into balls. Place on the prepared baking sheet.
5. Flatten each ball slightly with the back of a spoon or your fingers.
6. Bake for 12-15 minutes, or until macaroons are golden brown around the edges.
7. Remove from the oven and let cool on the baking sheet for 5 minutes.
8. Transfer macaroons to a wire rack to cool completely.
9. If desired, drizzle melted dark chocolate over the cooled macaroons.
10. Let chocolate set before serving.
11. Serve as chewy and coconutty coconut macaroons.

8. Mango Coconut Chia Pudding

Ingredients:
- 1/4 cup chia seeds
- 1 cup coconut milk (unsweetened)
- 1 tablespoon honey or maple syrup
- 1/2 teaspoon vanilla extract
- 1 ripe mango, peeled and diced
- Toasted coconut flakes, for garnish (optional)

Instructions:
1. In a mixing bowl, combine chia seeds, coconut milk, honey or maple syrup, and vanilla extract.
2. Stir well to combine.
3. Cover and refrigerate for at least 2 hours or overnight, until the mixture thickens to a pudding-like consistency.
4. Stir the chia seed pudding before serving to ensure even texture.
5. Spoon chia seed pudding into serving bowls or glasses.
6. Top with diced ripe mango.
7. Sprinkle with toasted coconut flakes for added crunch and flavor, if desired.
8. Serve chilled as a tropical and creamy mango coconut chia pudding.

9. Greek Yogurt with Honey and Walnuts

Ingredients:
- 1 cup Greek yogurt (plain or vanilla, low-fat)
- 2 tablespoons honey
- 1/4 cup chopped walnuts
- Fresh berries, for garnish

Instructions:
1. Spoon Greek yogurt into serving bowls.
2. Drizzle honey over the yogurt.
3. Sprinkle chopped walnuts on top.
4. Garnish with fresh berries.
5. Serve immediately as a simple and protein-packed Greek yogurt with honey and walnuts.

10. Banana Ice Cream

Ingredients:
- 3 ripe bananas, peeled and sliced
- 1/4 cup almond milk or coconut milk (unsweetened)
- 1 teaspoon vanilla extract
- Dark chocolate chips or cocoa nibs (optional, for topping)

Instructions:
1. Place sliced ripe bananas on a parchment-lined baking sheet.
2. Freeze bananas for at least 2 hours or until solid.
3. In a food processor or blender, combine frozen banana slices, almond milk or coconut milk, and vanilla extract.
4. Blend until smooth and creamy, scraping down the sides as needed.
5. If desired, add dark chocolate chips or cocoa nibs during the last few seconds of blending for added texture.
6. Transfer banana ice cream to serving bowls.
7. Serve immediately as a guilt-free and naturally sweet banana ice cream.

11. Baked Pears with Honey and Cinnamon

Ingredients:
- 4 ripe pears, halved and cored
- 2 tablespoons honey
- 1 teaspoon ground cinnamon
- 1/4 cup chopped nuts (such as almonds or walnuts), for topping
- Greek yogurt or vanilla ice cream (optional, for serving)

Instructions:
1. Preheat the oven to 375°F (190°C). Line a baking dish with parchment paper.
2. Place halved and cored pears cut-side up in the baking dish.
3. Drizzle honey evenly over the pears.
4. Sprinkle ground cinnamon over the pears.
5. Bake for 25-30 minutes, or until pears are tender and caramelized.
6. Remove from the oven and let cool slightly.
7. Sprinkle chopped nuts over the baked pears.
8. Serve warm with a dollop of Greek yogurt or a scoop of vanilla ice cream, if desired.
9. Enjoy these simple and naturally sweet baked pears with honey and cinnamon.

12. Blueberry Chia Seed Jam

Ingredients:
- 2 cups fresh or frozen blueberries
- 2 tablespoons chia seeds
- 1 tablespoon honey or maple syrup (optional, adjust to taste)
- 1 tablespoon lemon juice

Instructions:
1. In a saucepan, combine blueberries and lemon juice.
2. Cook over medium heat, stirring occasionally, until blueberries start to break down and release their juices, about 5-7 minutes.
3. Mash the blueberries with a fork or potato masher to desired consistency.
4. Stir in chia seeds and honey or maple syrup (if using).

5. Continue to cook for another 5-7 minutes, stirring frequently, until the mixture thickens.
6. Remove from heat and let cool.
7. Transfer blueberry chia seed jam to a jar or container.
8. Refrigerate for at least 1 hour to allow the jam to set.
9. Serve chilled as a delicious and nutrient-packed blueberry chia seed jam.

13. Pumpkin Spice Baked Oatmeal Cups

Ingredients:
- 2 cups rolled oats (gluten-free if needed)
- 1 teaspoon baking powder
- 1/2 teaspoon ground cinnamon
- 1/4 teaspoon ground nutmeg
- 1/4 teaspoon ground ginger
- 1/4 teaspoon salt
- 1 cup pumpkin puree
- 1/2 cup milk (dairy or non-dairy)
- 1/4 cup honey or maple syrup
- 1 teaspoon vanilla extract
- 1/4 cup chopped pecans or walnuts (optional)

Instructions:
1. Preheat the oven to 350°F (175°C). Grease a muffin tin or line with paper liners.
2. In a large bowl, combine rolled oats, baking powder, ground cinnamon, ground nutmeg, ground ginger, and salt.
3. In another bowl, whisk together pumpkin puree, milk, honey or maple syrup, and vanilla extract until smooth.
4. Pour wet ingredients into dry ingredients and stir until well combined.
5. Fold in chopped pecans or walnuts, if using.
6. Spoon oatmeal mixture into the prepared muffin tin, filling each cup to the top.
7. Bake for 20-25 minutes, or until oatmeal cups are set and lightly golden.
8. Remove from the oven and let cool in the muffin tin for 5 minutes.
9. Transfer oatmeal cups to a wire rack to cool completely.

10. Serve warm or at room temperature as wholesome and pumpkin-spiced baked oatmeal cups.

14. Fruit Salad with Citrus Dressing

Ingredients:
- 2 cups mixed fresh fruit (such as strawberries, kiwi, oranges, grapes)
- 1 tablespoon honey or maple syrup
- 1 tablespoon fresh lemon juice
- Zest of 1 lemon
- Fresh mint leaves, for garnish

Instructions:
1. In a large bowl, combine mixed fresh fruit.
2. In a small bowl, whisk together honey or maple syrup, fresh lemon juice, and lemon zest.
3. Pour citrus dressing over the mixed fresh fruit and gently toss to coat.
4. Garnish with fresh mint leaves.
5. Serve chilled as a refreshing and colorful fruit salad with citrus dressing.

15. Apple Cinnamon Baked Quinoa

Ingredients:
- 1 cup quinoa, rinsed
- 2 cups water or almond milk (unsweetened)
- 2 apples, peeled and diced
- 1/4 cup raisins or dried cranberries
- 1 teaspoon ground cinnamon
- 1/4 teaspoon ground nutmeg
- 1/4 teaspoon salt
- 2 tablespoons honey or maple syrup

Instructions:
1. Preheat the oven to 350°F (175°C). Grease a baking dish with olive oil or coconut oil.

2. In a saucepan, combine quinoa and water or almond milk. Bring to a boil.
3. Reduce heat to low, cover, and simmer for 15 minutes, or until quinoa is cooked and liquid is absorbed.
4. In a large bowl, combine cooked quinoa, diced apples, raisins or dried cranberries, ground cinnamon, ground nutmeg, salt, and honey or maple syrup.
5. Stir well to combine all ingredients.
6. Transfer quinoa mixture to the greased baking dish.
7. Bake for 20-25 minutes, or until the apples are tender and the quinoa is lightly golden on top.
8. Remove from the oven and let cool slightly before serving.
9. Serve warm as a comforting and nutrient-rich apple cinnamon baked quinoa.

16. Lemon Poppy Seed Energy Balls

Ingredients:
- 1 cup rolled oats (gluten-free if needed)
- 1/2 cup almond butter or sunflower seed butter
- 1/4 cup honey or maple syrup
- Zest of 1 lemon
- Juice of 1/2 lemon
- 2 tablespoons poppy seeds
- Pinch of salt

Instructions:
1. In a food processor, combine rolled oats, almond butter or sunflower seed butter, honey or maple syrup, lemon zest, lemon juice, poppy seeds, and a pinch of salt.
2. Pulse until mixture comes together and forms a sticky dough.
3. Scoop tablespoon-sized portions of the dough and roll into balls using your hands.
4. Place energy balls on a parchment-lined baking sheet.
5. Refrigerate for 30 minutes to set.
6. Serve chilled as zesty and nutrient-packed lemon poppy seed energy balls.

17. Cocoa Almond Butter Banana Bites

Ingredients:
- 2 ripe bananas, peeled and sliced
- 2 tablespoons almond butter or peanut butter
- 2 tablespoons unsweetened cocoa powder
- 1/4 cup chopped almonds or walnuts
- Dark chocolate chips (optional, for topping)

Instructions:
1. Lay banana slices flat on a parchment-lined baking sheet.
2. Spread almond butter or peanut butter over half of the banana slices.
3. Dust the remaining banana slices with unsweetened cocoa powder.
4. Sandwich together banana slices to form bites.
5. Press chopped almonds or walnuts onto the sides of the banana bites.
6. If desired, melt dark chocolate chips and drizzle over the banana bites for added indulgence.
7. Refrigerate for 30 minutes to set.
8. Serve chilled as creamy and chocolaty cocoa almond butter banana bites.

18. Date and Nut Bars

Ingredients:
- 1 cup pitted dates, chopped
- 1 cup mixed nuts (such as almonds, cashews, pecans), chopped
- 1/4 cup unsweetened shredded coconut
- 1/4 cup almond butter or cashew butter
- 1 tablespoon honey or maple syrup
- Pinch of salt

Instructions:
1. In a food processor, combine chopped dates, mixed nuts, unsweetened shredded coconut, almond butter or cashew butter, honey or maple syrup, and a pinch of salt.
2. Pulse until mixture sticks together and forms a sticky dough.

3. Line a baking dish with parchment paper, leaving some overhang for easy removal.
4. Press date and nut mixture evenly into the baking dish.
5. Refrigerate for 1-2 hours, or until firm.
6. Remove from the refrigerator and lift bars out of the baking dish using the parchment paper overhang.
7. Cut into bars or squares.
8. Serve chilled or at room temperature as nutritious and naturally sweet date and nut bars.

19. Carrot Cake Energy Bites

Ingredients:
- 1 cup rolled oats (gluten-free if needed)
- 1/2 cup grated carrots
- 1/4 cup almond butter or sunflower seed butter
- 1/4 cup honey or maple syrup
- 1 teaspoon ground cinnamon
- 1/2 teaspoon ground nutmeg
- 1/4 cup chopped walnuts or pecans
- Unsweetened shredded coconut (optional, for rolling)

Instructions:
1. In a mixing bowl, combine rolled oats, grated carrots, almond butter or sunflower seed butter, honey or maple syrup, ground cinnamon, ground nutmeg, and chopped walnuts or pecans.
2. Stir until well combined and the mixture holds together.
3. Scoop tablespoon-sized portions of the mixture and roll into balls using your hands.
4. Optional: Roll energy bites in unsweetened shredded coconut for extra texture and flavor.
5. Refrigerate for 30 minutes to set.
6. Serve chilled as carrot cake-inspired and nutrient-packed energy bites.

20. Vanilla Almond Chia Pudding

Ingredients:
- 1/4 cup chia seeds
- 1 cup almond milk (unsweetened)
- 1 tablespoon honey or maple syrup
- 1/2 teaspoon vanilla extract
- Sliced almonds, for topping

Instructions:
1. In a mixing bowl, combine chia seeds, almond milk, honey or maple syrup, and vanilla extract.
2. Stir well to combine.
3. Cover and refrigerate for at least 2 hours or overnight, until the mixture thickens to a pudding-like consistency.
4. Stir the chia seed pudding before serving to ensure even texture.
5. Spoon chia seed pudding into serving bowls or glasses.
6. Top with sliced almonds.
7. Serve chilled as a creamy and subtly sweet vanilla almond chia pudding.

9. 28-Day Meal Plan

Week 1 Shopping List

Produce:
- Avocados
- Eggs
- Quinoa
- Mixed vegetables (such as bell peppers, zucchini, broccoli)
- Spinach
- Mushrooms
- Tomatoes
- Cucumbers
- Carrots
- Lemons
- Berries (blueberries, strawberries, raspberries)
- Apples
- Mango
- Fresh herbs (such as basil, parsley, mint)
- Bananas

Proteins:
- Salmon filets
- Chicken breasts
- Ground turkey or chicken
- Shrimp
- Canned chickpeas
- Canned lentils
- Tuna (canned or fresh)

Dairy and Alternatives:
- Greek yogurt
- Almond milk (unsweetened)

Grains and Breads:

- Whole grain bread
- Brown rice
- Whole wheat pasta (optional)
- Rolled oats
- Almond flour (for pancakes)

Nuts and Seeds:
- Almonds
- Walnuts
- Chia seeds
- Poppy seeds

Pantry Staples:
- Olive oil
- Coconut oil
- Honey or maple syrup
- Balsamic vinegar
- Low-sodium soy sauce or tamari
- Dijon mustard
- Spices and seasonings (cinnamon, nutmeg, ginger, salt, pepper)

Desserts:
- Dark chocolate chips
- Dates
- Unsweetened shredded coconut
- Cocoa powder

Week 1 Recipes

Day 1:
- Breakfast: Avocado Toast with Poached Egg
- Lunch: Quinoa Salad with Roasted Vegetables
- Dinner: Baked Salmon with Steamed Broccoli
- Snack: Greek Yogurt with Berries
- Dessert: Dark Chocolate Covered Strawberries

Day 2:
- Breakfast: Blueberry Chia Seed Smoothie
- Lunch: Mediterranean Chickpea Salad
- Dinner: Turkey Meatballs with Zucchini Noodles
- Snack: Carrot Sticks with Hummus
- Dessert: Date and Nut Bars

Day 3:
- Breakfast: Pumpkin Spice Baked Oatmeal Cups
- Lunch: Lentil Soup with Whole Grain Bread
- Dinner: Chicken Stir-Fry with Brown Rice
- Snack: Apple Slices with Almond Butter
- Dessert: Banana Chia Pudding

Day 4:
- Breakfast: Greek Yogurt Parfait with Granola and Mixed Berries
- Lunch: Spinach and Mushroom Quiche
- Dinner: Beef and Vegetable Stew
- Snack: Date and Nut Bars
- Dessert: Cocoa Almond Butter Banana Bites

Day 5:
- Breakfast: Mango Coconut Chia Pudding
- Lunch: Caprese Salad with Grilled Chicken
- Dinner: Stuffed Bell Peppers with Ground Turkey and Quinoa
- Snack: Cocoa Almond Butter Banana Bites
- Dessert: Dark Chocolate Energy Balls

Day 6:
- Breakfast: Almond Flour Pancakes with Fresh Fruit
- Lunch: Tuna Salad Lettuce Wraps
- Dinner: Grilled Shrimp Skewers with Quinoa Salad
- Snack: Lemon Poppy Seed Energy Balls
- Dessert: Coconut Date Rolls

Day 7:
- Breakfast: Overnight Oats with Berries and Almonds
- Lunch: Greek Chicken Salad
- Dinner: Vegetable Curry with Cauliflower Rice
- Snack: Greek Yogurt with Honey and Walnuts
- Dessert: Banana Almond Butter Bites

Week 2 Shopping List

Produce:
- Avocados
- Eggs
- Quinoa
- Mixed vegetables (such as bell peppers, zucchini, broccoli)
- Spinach
- Mushrooms
- Tomatoes
- Cucumbers
- Carrots
- Lemons
- Berries (blueberries, strawberries, raspberries)
- Apples
- Mango
- Fresh herbs (such as basil, parsley, mint)
- Bananas

Proteins:
- Salmon filets
- Chicken breasts
- Ground turkey or chicken
- Shrimp
- Canned chickpeas
- Canned lentils
- Tuna (canned or fresh)

Dairy and Alternatives:
- Greek yogurt
- Almond milk (unsweetened)

Grains and Breads:
- Whole grain bread
- Brown rice

- Whole wheat pasta (optional)
- Rolled oats
- Almond flour (for pancakes)

Nuts and Seeds:
- Almonds
- Walnuts
- Chia seeds
- Poppy seeds

Pantry Staples:
- Olive oil
- Coconut oil
- Honey or maple syrup
- Balsamic vinegar
- Low-sodium soy sauce or tamari
- Dijon mustard
- Spices and seasonings (cinnamon, nutmeg, ginger, salt, pepper)

Desserts:
- Dark chocolate chips
- Dates
- Unsweetened shredded coconut
- Cocoa powder

Week 2 Recipes

Day 8:
- Breakfast: Avocado Toast with Poached Egg
- Lunch: Quinoa Salad with Roasted Vegetables
- Dinner: Baked Salmon with Steamed Broccoli
- Snack: Greek Yogurt with Berries
- Dessert: Dark Chocolate Covered Strawberries

Day 9:
- Breakfast: Blueberry Chia Seed Smoothie
- Lunch: Mediterranean Chickpea Salad
- Dinner: Turkey Meatballs with Zucchini Noodles
- Snack: Carrot Sticks with Hummus
- Dessert: Date and Nut Bars

Day 10:
- Breakfast: Pumpkin Spice Baked Oatmeal Cups
- Lunch: Lentil Soup with Whole Grain Bread
- Dinner: Chicken Stir-Fry with Brown Rice
- Snack: Apple Slices with Almond Butter
- Dessert: Banana Chia Pudding

Day 11:
- Breakfast: Greek Yogurt Parfait with Granola and Mixed Berries
- Lunch: Spinach and Mushroom Quiche
- Dinner: Beef and Vegetable Stew
- Snack: Date and Nut Bars
- Dessert: Cocoa Almond Butter Banana Bites

Day 12:
- Breakfast: Mango Coconut Chia Pudding
- Lunch: Caprese Salad with Grilled Chicken
- Dinner: Stuffed Bell Peppers with Ground Turkey and Quinoa
- Snack: Cocoa Almond Butter Banana Bites
- Dessert: Dark Chocolate Energy Balls

Day 13:
- Breakfast: Almond Flour Pancakes with Fresh Fruit
- Lunch: Tuna Salad Lettuce Wraps
- Dinner: Grilled Shrimp Skewers with Quinoa Salad
- Snack: Lemon Poppy Seed Energy Balls
- Dessert: Coconut Date Rolls

Day 14:
- Breakfast: Overnight Oats with Berries and Almonds
- Lunch: Greek Chicken Salad
- Dinner: Vegetable Curry with Cauliflower Rice
- Snack: Greek Yogurt with Honey and Walnuts
- Dessert: Banana Almond Butter Bites

Week 3 Shopping List

Produce:
- Avocados
- Eggs
- Quinoa
- Mixed vegetables (such as bell peppers, zucchini, broccoli)
- Spinach
- Mushrooms
- Tomatoes
- Cucumbers
- Carrots
- Lemons
- Berries (blueberries, strawberries, raspberries)
- Apples
- Mango
- Fresh herbs (such as basil, parsley, mint)
- Bananas

Proteins:
- Salmon filets
- Chicken breasts
- Ground turkey or chicken
- Shrimp
- Canned chickpeas
- Canned lentils
- Tuna (canned or fresh)

Dairy and Alternatives:
- Greek yogurt
- Almond milk (unsweetened)

Grains and Breads:
- Whole grain bread
- Brown rice

- Whole wheat pasta (optional)
- Rolled oats
- Almond flour (for pancakes)

Nuts and Seeds:
- Almonds
- Walnuts
- Chia seeds
- Poppy seeds

Pantry Staples:
- Olive oil
- Coconut oil
- Honey or maple syrup
- Balsamic vinegar
- Low-sodium soy sauce or tamari
- Dijon mustard
- Spices and seasonings (cinnamon, nutmeg, ginger, salt, pepper)

Desserts:
- Dark chocolate chips
- Dates
- Unsweetened shredded coconut
- Cocoa powder

Week 3 Recipes

Day 15:
- Breakfast: Avocado Toast with Poached Egg
- Lunch: Quinoa Salad with Roasted Vegetables
- Dinner: Baked Salmon with Steamed Broccoli
- Snack: Greek Yogurt with Berries
- Dessert: Dark Chocolate Covered Strawberries

Day 16:
- Breakfast: Blueberry Chia Seed Smoothie
- Lunch: Mediterranean Chickpea Salad
- Dinner: Turkey Meatballs with Zucchini Noodles
- Snack: Carrot Sticks with Hummus
- Dessert: Date and Nut Bars

Day 17:
- Breakfast: Pumpkin Spice Baked Oatmeal Cups
- Lunch: Lentil Soup with Whole Grain Bread
- Dinner: Chicken Stir-Fry with Brown Rice
- Snack: Apple Slices with Almond Butter
- Dessert: Banana Chia Pudding

Day 18:
- Breakfast: Greek Yogurt Parfait with Granola and Mixed Berries
- Lunch: Spinach and Mushroom Quiche
- Dinner: Beef and Vegetable Stew
- Snack: Date and Nut Bars
- Dessert: Cocoa Almond Butter Banana Bites

Day 19:
- Breakfast: Mango Coconut Chia Pudding
- Lunch: Caprese Salad with Grilled Chicken
- Dinner: Stuffed Bell Peppers with Ground Turkey and Quinoa
- Snack: Cocoa Almond Butter Banana Bites
- Dessert: Dark Chocolate Energy Balls

Day 20:
- Breakfast: Almond Flour Pancakes with Fresh Fruit
- Lunch: Tuna Salad Lettuce Wraps
- Dinner: Grilled Shrimp Skewers with Quinoa Salad
- Snack: Lemon Poppy Seed Energy Balls
- Dessert: Coconut Date Rolls

Day 21:
- Breakfast: Overnight Oats with Berries and Almonds
- Lunch: Greek Chicken Salad
- Dinner: Vegetable Curry with Cauliflower Rice
- Snack: Greek Yogurt with Honey and Walnuts
- Dessert: Banana Almond Butter Bites

Week 4 Shopping List

Produce:
- Avocados
- Eggs
- Quinoa
- Mixed vegetables (such as bell peppers, zucchini, broccoli)
- Spinach
- Mushrooms
- Tomatoes
- Cucumbers
- Carrots
- Lemons
- Berries (blueberries, strawberries, raspberries)
- Apples
- Mango
- Fresh herbs (such as basil, parsley, mint)
- Bananas

Proteins:
- Salmon filets
- Chicken breasts
- Ground turkey or chicken
- Shrimp
- Canned chickpeas
- Canned lentils
- Tuna (canned or fresh)

Dairy and Alternatives:
- Greek yogurt
- Almond milk (unsweetened)

Grains and Breads:
- Whole grain bread
- Brown rice

- Whole wheat pasta (optional)
- Rolled oats
- Almond flour (for pancakes)

Nuts and Seeds:
- Almonds
- Walnuts
- Chia seeds
- Poppy seeds

Pantry Staples:
- Olive oil
- Coconut oil
- Honey or maple syrup
- Balsamic vinegar
- Low-sodium soy sauce or tamari
- Dijon mustard
- Spices and seasonings (cinnamon, nutmeg, ginger, salt, pepper)

Desserts:
- Dark chocolate chips
- Dates
- Unsweetened shredded coconut
- Cocoa powder

Week 4 Recipes

Day 22:
- Breakfast: Avocado Toast with Poached Egg
- Lunch: Quinoa Salad with Roasted Vegetables
- Dinner: Baked Salmon with Steamed Broccoli
- Snack: Greek Yogurt with Berries
- Dessert: Dark Chocolate Covered Strawberries

Day 23:
- Breakfast: Blueberry Chia Seed Smoothie
- Lunch: Mediterranean Chickpea Salad
- Dinner: Turkey Meatballs with Zucchini Noodles
- Snack: Carrot Sticks with Hummus
- Dessert: Date and Nut Bars

Day 24:
- Breakfast: Pumpkin Spice Baked Oatmeal Cups
- Lunch: Lentil Soup with Whole Grain Bread
- Dinner: Chicken Stir-Fry with Brown Rice
- Snack: Apple Slices with Almond Butter
- Dessert: Banana Chia Pudding

Day 25:
- Breakfast: Greek Yogurt Parfait with Granola and Mixed Berries
- Lunch: Spinach and Mushroom Quiche
- Dinner: Beef and Vegetable Stew
- Snack: Date and Nut Bars
- Dessert: Cocoa Almond Butter Banana Bites

Day 26:
- Breakfast: Mango Coconut Chia Pudding
- Lunch: Caprese Salad with Grilled Chicken
- Dinner: Stuffed Bell Peppers with Ground Turkey and Quinoa
- Snack: Cocoa Almond Butter Banana Bites
- Dessert: Dark Chocolate Energy Balls

Day 27:
- Breakfast: Almond Flour Pancakes with Fresh Fruit
- Lunch: Tuna Salad Lettuce Wraps
- Dinner: Grilled Shrimp Skewers with Quinoa Salad
- Snack: Lemon Poppy Seed Energy Balls
- Dessert: Coconut Date Rolls

Day 28:
- Breakfast: Overnight Oats with Berries and Almonds
- Lunch: Greek Chicken Salad
- Dinner: Vegetable Curry with Cauliflower Rice
- Snack: Greek Yogurt with Honey and Walnuts
- Dessert: Banana Almond Butter Bites

10. Lifestyle Tips

Hydration and Brain Health

Staying hydrated is crucial for overall health, but it's especially important for brain function. The brain is about 75% water, and even mild dehydration can impair cognitive function, mood, and energy levels. For individuals newly diagnosed with Alzheimer's, maintaining proper hydration can support better brain health and potentially slow cognitive decline. Here are some tips to ensure you stay well-hydrated:

1. Drink Plenty of Water: Aim for at least 8 cups (64 ounces) of water per day. This can vary based on individual needs, activity level, and climate.
2. Set Reminders: If remembering to drink water is challenging, set regular reminders on your phone or use a hydration tracking app.
3. Infuse Your Water: If plain water is unappealing, try adding slices of fruits like lemon, lime, or berries, or herbs like mint to make it more enjoyable.
4. Eat Hydrating Foods: Incorporate foods with high water content into your diet, such as cucumbers, tomatoes, watermelon, and oranges.
5. Limit Dehydrating Beverages: Reduce intake of alcohol and caffeine, as they can contribute to dehydration. If you do consume these, balance with extra water.
6. Monitor Urine Color: A simple way to check hydration is by the color of your urine. Light yellow usually indicates good hydration, while dark yellow suggests you need to drink more fluids.
7. Stay Consistent: Drink water consistently throughout the day rather than trying to meet your hydration needs all at once.

By incorporating these hydration tips into your daily routine, you can help support brain health and overall well-being.

Physical Activity and Cognitive Function

Engaging in regular physical activity is another essential component of maintaining cognitive health, especially for those newly diagnosed with Alzheimer's. Exercise promotes blood flow to the brain, supports the growth of new neurons, and can improve mood and sleep. Here are some tips to help incorporate physical activity into your routine:

1. Aim for Consistency: Try to be active most days of the week, aiming for at least 150 minutes of moderate-intensity aerobic activity, such as brisk walking, per week.
2. Include Strength Training: Incorporate strength training exercises at least two days a week to help maintain muscle mass and overall strength. This can include activities like lifting weights, using resistance bands, or body-weight exercises.
3. Find Enjoyable Activities: Choose exercises you enjoy to make it easier to stick with your routine. This could be dancing, swimming, cycling, gardening, or yoga.
4. Stay Social: Join exercise classes or walking groups to make physical activity a social event. Engaging with others can also provide emotional support and motivation.
5. Incorporate Balance and Flexibility Exercises: Activities such as yoga and tai chi can improve balance and flexibility, which are important for overall physical function and can reduce the risk of falls.
6. Set Realistic Goals: Start with small, achievable goals and gradually increase the intensity and duration of your activities as your fitness improves.
7. Stay Safe: Ensure that any exercise routine is safe and appropriate for your current fitness level. Consult with a healthcare professional before starting a new exercise program, especially if you have any other health conditions.
8. Listen to Your Body: Pay attention to how your body feels during and after exercise. It's important to push yourself, but not to the point of pain or excessive fatigue.

By making physical activity a regular part of your lifestyle, you can enhance cognitive function, improve physical health, and boost your overall quality of life.

Stress Management and Sleep

Managing stress and ensuring adequate sleep are critical components of maintaining cognitive health, especially for those newly diagnosed with Alzheimer's. Chronic stress and poor sleep can negatively impact brain function and overall well-being. Here are some tips for managing stress and improving sleep quality:

1. Establish a Sleep Routine: Go to bed and wake up at the same time every day, even on weekends. This helps regulate your body's internal clock.

2. Create a Relaxing Bedtime Routine: Engage in calming activities before bed, such as reading, taking a warm bath, or practicing relaxation techniques like deep breathing or meditation.

3. Limit Screen Time: Reduce exposure to screens (phones, tablets, TVs) at least an hour before bedtime, as the blue light emitted can interfere with your sleep cycle.

4. Create a Comfortable Sleep Environment: Ensure your bedroom is conducive to sleep by keeping it cool, dark, and quiet. Consider using earplugs or a white noise machine if needed.

5. Be Mindful of Food and Drink: Avoid large meals, caffeine, and alcohol close to bedtime, as they can disrupt sleep.

6. Exercise Regularly: Regular physical activity can help you fall asleep faster and enjoy deeper sleep. Just avoid vigorous exercise close to bedtime.

7. Practice Stress Management Techniques: Incorporate stress-reducing practices into your daily routine, such as mindfulness meditation, yoga, deep breathing exercises, or journaling.

8. Stay Connected: Maintain social connections and engage in activities you enjoy. Social interaction can help reduce feelings of isolation and stress.

9. Seek Professional Help: If you're struggling with managing stress or sleep issues, consider speaking with a healthcare professional. They can provide personalized strategies and support.

10. Mindfulness and Relaxation: Practices such as mindfulness meditation, progressive muscle relaxation, and guided imagery can help calm the mind and reduce stress.

11. Stay Positive: Focus on positive aspects of life and practice gratitude. Keeping a gratitude journal can be a simple yet effective way to shift your mindset and reduce stress.

By incorporating these tips into your daily routine, you can better manage stress and improve sleep quality, both of which are essential for maintaining cognitive health and overall well-being.

11. Conclusion

Navigating the journey of an Alzheimer's diagnosis can be daunting and overwhelming. However, it is important to remember that you are not alone. This cookbook and guide is designed to be a supportive companion, offering practical and compassionate advice to help you manage this new chapter in your life.

Each recipe, tip, and piece of advice has been carefully selected with your health and well-being in mind. Our goal is to provide you with the tools you need to nourish not only your body but also your mind and spirit. The connection between diet, lifestyle, and cognitive health is profound, and by making thoughtful choices, you can positively impact your journey with Alzheimer's.

We understand that every day may bring different challenges, but it also brings new opportunities to care for yourself and those you love. Embrace each meal as a step towards better health and a moment of mindfulness. Celebrate the small victories, whether it's mastering a new recipe, enjoying a walk in the park, or simply sharing a meal with loved ones.

Remember to be kind to yourself. This journey is not just about managing a condition, but also about living a life filled with moments of joy, connection, and fulfillment. Reach out for support when you need it, and cherish the support network around you.

As you turn the pages of this cookbook, let it remind you that every effort you make towards a healthier lifestyle is a testament to your strength and resilience. You are taking important steps to nurture your body and mind, and that is something truly remarkable.

We hope that this guide serves as a beacon of hope, encouragement, and empowerment. May it inspire you to explore new flavors, enjoy wholesome meals, and embrace a lifestyle that supports your cognitive health and overall well-being. Together, we can face the challenges and celebrate the triumphs, one meal at a time.

www.ingramcontent.com/pod-product-compliance
Lightning Source LLC
Chambersburg PA
CBHW082237220526
45479CB00005B/1257